CHILDREN'

CHILDREN'S HOMES

A History of Institutional Care for Britain's Young

Peter Higginbotham

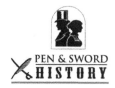

PEN & SWORD HISTORY

For my mother

First published in Great Britain in 2017 and reprinted in 2022 by
Pen & Sword History
an imprint of
Pen & Sword Books Ltd
47 Church Street
Barnsley
South Yorkshire
S70 2AS

ISBN 978 1 52670 135 0

A CIP catalogue record for this book is
available from the British Library.

Printed and bound in England
By CPI Group (UK) Ltd, Croydon, CR0 4YY

Pen & Sword Books Ltd incorporates the Imprints of Pen & Sword Books
Archaeology, Atlas, Aviation, Battleground, Discovery, Family History, History,
Maritime, Military, Naval, Politics, Railways, Select, Transport, True Crime,
Fiction, Frontline Books, Leo Cooper, Praetorian Press, Seaforth Publishing,
Wharncliffe and White Owl.

For a complete list of Pen & Sword titles please contact
PEN & SWORD BOOKS LIMITED
47 Church Street, Barnsley, South Yorkshire, S70 2AS, England
E-mail: enquiries@pen-and-sword.co.uk
Website: www.pen-and-sword.co.uk

Contents

Introduction

What image does the word 'orphanage' conjure up in your mind? A sunny scene of carefree children at play in the grounds of a large ivy-clad house? Or a forbidding grey edifice whose cowering inmates are ruled over with a rod of iron by a stern, starched matron? Ever since Victorian times, the promotional and fund-raising literature for children's homes has, of course, tried to portray them as rather idyllic places where, despite their unfortunate situations, the residents were tenderly nurtured. However, there is now much evidence that some children's institutions were indeed fearful places where children were, at least by present-day standards, badly treated – even if it was often with the best of intentions by those who ran those establishments. Events in more recent times have given us an even grimmer image of children's homes as places where the residents were sometimes subjected to horrendous physical and sexual abuse by those in whose care they had been placed. So what is the real story? Who founded and ran all these institutions? Who paid for them? Where have they all gone? And what was life like for their inmates?

Over the years, children have needed to find residential care outside their own family for many and diverse reasons. Orphans – those whose parents were both dead – were perhaps the most obvious group in need of a new home, but children in rather less clear-cut situations could also be included in this category. Children having just one available parent, sometimes referred to as 'partial' orphans, were often treated with the same regard as 'full' orphans, as were those whose parents had abandoned them.

Destitution, by reason of the parents' unemployment, illness or other circumstances, was another common cause of a child's needing care to be provided, although this might only be on a temporary basis if the parents' situation changed. By the middle of the nineteenth century, there was also increasing concern for children whose parents were considered unfit for the role, or where the home environment was deemed to be detrimental to the children's welfare.

Although institutional care for disadvantaged children can be traced back to at least Tudor times, it was the latter part of the eighteenth century that saw the rise of charitably funded 'asylums' for the orphaned or destitute, particularly in London. The number of these gradually increased, with establishments also being founded for the children of soldiers, mariners, police officers, railway workers and other occupations. However, it was not until the last quarter of the nineteenth century that the voluntary provision of institutional care for the young became widely available. Up until that time, for most children in difficult circumstances, it was the workhouse only that had offered an alternative home.

Much of the activity that resulted in this new provision was by groups who believed that children needed to be 'rescued' from bad surroundings and placed in institutional care, where they could be given the education, practical training, discipline and, above all, the religious instruction that would stand them in good stead in their adult lives. The Victorian period also witnessed an expansion of the middle class who provided considerable support for the increasing number of charitable organizations. This included not only direct financial contributions, but also a veritable army of women, often well educated, with the time and resources to assist charities in their administration and fund-raising efforts.

In both the charitable and workhouse sectors, the physical form taken by their children's provision evolved considerably over the years, gradually moving away from large monolithic orphanage institutions to the much more domestic scale of 'cottage homes' and 'family group' accommodation. For boys with an interest in a seafaring career, a number of training ships were set up.

Concern that children from particular religious communities should not be in danger of losing their faith, particularly when placed in the workhouse environment, led to the setting up of many homes by religious organizations, most notably the Roman Catholic Church. Such groups were also frequently involved in the increasing provision of 'preventive' homes for girls in moral danger, and Penitentiaries or Magdalen Homes for young, unmarried mothers.

Special homes were set up, too, for children with a variety of physical or mental disabilities, and diseases such as tuberculosis, together with convalescent homes for children who were frail or recovering from illness.

In the 1850s, for children who had committed a criminal offence, an alternative to prison became available to the courts in the shape of the Reformatory School. For those discovered sleeping rough, or who were considered in moral danger, or beyond their parents' control, the Industrial School – an evolution of the Ragged School – formalized the process of what we would now refer to as being taken into care. In the 1930s, the Reformatory and Industrial Schools were replaced by Approved Schools, themselves succeeded in the 1970s by Community Homes with Education.

For organizations which took children into care on a permanent basis, there could never be enough places for all those who came their way. To keep the door open to new arrivals, the ongoing 'disposal' of at least some of their existing charges was a constant concern. Two main solutions were adopted for dealing with this problem. The first was boarding out – what we now call fostering – where children were placed with families who received a weekly payment to cover the costs. The second was emigration, where large numbers of children were sent to begin new lives overseas, with Canada being the main destination until the 1920s when Australia became a more amenable host. Homes were established in Britain to prepare those about to emigrate, and in Canada and Australia to receive new arrivals before they were dispersed to their new families or employers.

After the Second World War, local authorities were given the leading role in the provision of children's services. At the same time, the focus of children's care underwent a major shift away from institutional accommodation towards fostering. These developments, together with changing social attitudes towards matters such as single motherhood, led to a steady decline in the demand for residential places in the voluntary sector. By the 1980s, virtually all the homes run by the traditional children's charities had closed. The central role of local authorities as the front-line provider of children's services continues to the present day. Increasingly, however, they contract out their residential care provision to the commercial sector.

The total number of children's establishments that operated over the years runs into many thousands, and the children that lived in them probably into millions. Some homes were short-lived, while a few were around for the best part of a century. Many were run by large organizations, some by a single individual. Casting its net wide, this book takes a look at how these many and varied institutions operated and evolved in the context of changing views of how best to serve the needs of the children in their care.

Chapter 1

Early Children's Homes

Christ's Hospital

A strong claim to being England's first institutional home for poor or orphan children can be made by Christ's Hospital, which was situated on London's Newgate Street, a couple of hundred yards to the north of St Paul's Cathedral. The building, formerly the Greyfriars monastery, was a victim of Henry VIII's dissolution of England's religious houses. Henry subsequently made little use of the property and in December 1546 handed it over to the City of London to be used for relief of the poor. Having acquired Greyfriars, however, the City appears to have lost interest in its further development, perhaps lacking the necessary funds.

Four years later, after hearing an impassioned sermon by the Bishop of London, Nicholas Ridley, about the plight of London's poor, the young Edward VI confirmed his father's gift and, more importantly, provided the institution with an endowment of £600 a year. He commissioned the Lord Mayor of London, Sir Richard Dodd, to take the matter forward and a committee was formed to oversee the project and raise further funds. By November 1552, the buildings had been refurbished and 340 poor, fatherless children were admitted into what then became known as Christ's Hospital. The term 'hospital' at that time signified a place of refuge rather than a medical facility.

The uniform that came to be adopted for the inmates of the Hospital comprised a black cap, a long blue gown with a red belt, and yellow stockings. The colours were chosen for very practical reasons: blue was the colour obtained from a cheap dye and worn by servants and apprentices, while yellow was believed to discourage lice.[1] The institution soon gained the alternative name of the Blue Coat School, and its outfit was subsequently copied by other institutions that modelled themselves on Christ's, such as Queen Elizabeth's Hospital in Bristol (founded 1586), the Blue Coat School in Canterbury (1574), Lincoln Christ's Hospital School (1614), the Blue School in Wells (1641), the Reading Blue Coat School (1646) and Chetham's Hospital in Manchester (1652).

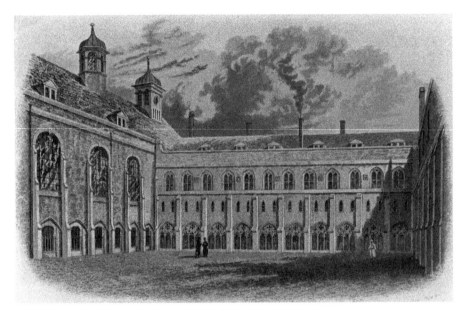

Part of Christ's Hospital in about 1700. After being severely damaged in the Great Fire of London, its rebuilding was completed in 1705 from designs by Sir Christopher Wren, a governor of the Hospital.

By the eighteenth century, the original London establishment was no longer housing the poorest children, but was boarding and educating 'the orphans of the lower clergy, officers and indigent gentlemen as could secure nomination by a member of the governing body'.[2] In 1902, the school moved to new premises near Horsham, Sussex, where it continues to the present day.

Bridewell

Bishop Ridley also persuaded Edward to give the City another royal property, a little-used former residence of Henry VIII on the banks of the River Fleet, known as Bridewell Palace. Bridewell took on a new lease of life at the end of 1556, with a role somewhere between that of a prison, a workhouse and a reformatory. Its inmates were primarily adults – vagrants, idlers and prostitutes – who, for a period ranging from a few weeks to several years, could be placed under its regime of daily labour and strict discipline. Bridewell's intake also included the young, however. The orphaned sons of City freemen were received there, parish officials sent destitute children, and the establishment's own beadles directed others from the streets to its doors.[3] As well as receiving a basic education, many of these children became apprentices in one of the numerous trades for which training was provided at the institution, including pin-making, silk and ribbon weaving, hemp dressing, glove-making and carpentry. In 1631, there were sixteen craftsmen teaching their trades to 106 apprentices.[4] A number of other towns such as Oxford, Salisbury, Gloucester and Ipswich also set up institutions modelled on Bridewell.

London Corporation of the Poor

In around 1650, almost a century after Bridewell opened its doors, London's first workhouses proper were set up by the city's Corporation of the Poor, which was given two confiscated royal properties – Heydon House in the Minories, and the Wardrobe building in Vintry. The Corporation's provision for the children in its care included the teaching of singing. A verse of one of the children's songs paints a very rosy picture of their treatment:

> *In filthy rags we clothed were*
> *In good warm Raiment now appear*
> *From Dunghill to King's Palace transferred,*
> *Where Education, wholesome Food,*
> *Meat, drink and Lodging, all that's good*
> *For Soul and Body, are so well prepared.*[5]

Following the Restoration in 1660, when Charles II reclaimed his estates, the Corporation ceased its activities. It was revived in 1698, however, and established a new workhouse on Bishopsgate Street where all the City's 'poor children, beggars, vagrants, and other idle and disorderly persons' were to be accommodated and employed. The 'poor children' included those whose family or friends could not support themselves, the children of soldiers and sailors who had died or become incapacitated in the service of the Crown, and petty criminals who might otherwise have ended up facing the gallows. The children, up to 400 in number, were taught to read and write and to cast accounts. They were also employed in tasks such as spinning wool and flax, winding silk, sewing, knitting, and making their own clothes or shoes. Their uniform, made of russet cloth, had a badge on its breast representing a poor boy and a sheep and the motto 'God's Providence is our Inheritance'.[6]

The Bishopsgate workhouse was a substantial edifice, some 400 feet long, and divided into two sections, the Steward's side, where the children were accommodated, and the Keeper's side, where the 'idle and disorderly' adults were confined. The cost of maintaining the children was mostly covered by payments from their home parish, with funds for the running of the establishment also coming from money raised by the Corporation, from private charities, and from income produced by the children's own labour.

Charity Schools

Following the example set by Christ's Hospital, a modest number of other Blue Coat institutions gradually appeared. In the early 1700s, however, a major expansion began to take place in the provision of schools for poor or orphan children, mostly funded by public subscription or private benefaction.

The growth of the charity school movement owed much to its promotion by the Society for Promoting Christian Knowledge (SPCK), founded in 1698 to 'spread practical Christianity among the godless poor'.[7] The provision of a Christian-based education for the poorest children was seen as a useful way to assist in this endeavour. The Society offered encouragement and advice for those wishing to set up schools, providing sample rules for their operation, and acting as a central co-ordinating body. The curriculum taught in the schools typically comprised reading and writing, plus casting accounts for the boys and sewing for the girls. It also aimed to remind the children of their lowly position in life and the duty and respect that they owed to their betters.

Supporting charity schools became a fashionable activity for the well-to-do and a large number were eventually opened, some notable examples being the Greenwich Blue Coat Girls' School (1700), the Nottingham Blue Coat School (1706), and the Liverpool Blue Coat School (1708). Others were founded in towns and villages all across the country; in 1792 it was reckoned that a total of 1,631 charity schools had been established since the Reformation.[8]

Although the majority of charity schools were day schools, some were residential, effectively operating as children's homes. Typical of these were York's two subscription charity Schools – the Blue Coat School for boys and Grey Coat School for girls – both founded by York Corporation in 1705 in association with the SPCK. The schools catered for orphans or children from poor, large families, and provided accommodation for forty boys and twenty girls between the ages of 7 and 12. They were taught reading, writing, basic arithmetic and were instructed in the catechism. The boys became apprenticed to tradesmen in the city, while the girls were prepared for domestic service.[9]

Conditions in the schools sometimes left much to be desired. In 1795, it was reported that the girls at the York Grey Coat School were consistently underfed and ill-treated, their appearance sickly and dejected, and their ignorance extreme. At the same date, children at the London Grey Coat Hospital were said to be utterly wretched from constant flogging and semi-starvation.[10]

The Foundling Hospital

A significant development in children's residential care came in 1739 when Captain Thomas Coram founded a new institution for the 'education and maintenance of exposed and deserted young children'. The Foundling Hospital, England's first charity devoted exclusively to children, opened its doors on 25 March 1741 in temporary premises in Hatton Garden.

Infants up to the age of two months could be deposited at the Hospital, with no information needing to be given about the mother's identity. Those handing over a baby were asked to leave a 'mark or token', such as a ribbon or scrap of material, by which they could identify the child at a future date if required. Infants accepted into the Hospital were baptized and named, then placed with a wet nurse in the country until the age of three. After returning to the Hospital, they were taught to read and 'brought up to labour to fit their age and sex'.[11] At the age of 14, boys were apprenticed into a trade or went to sea. At 16, the girls were placed in domestic service, with some entering into employment at the Hospital.

In September 1742, the foundation stone was laid for the Hospital's new premises in Bloomsbury Fields to the west of Gray's Inn Lane. The 56-acre, green-field site, part of the Earl of Salisbury's estate, cost £6,500, the Earl giving the Hospital a £500 discount on the land's market value. The new building was intended to accommodate up to 400 children.

Demand for places at the Hospital rapidly exceeded the number available. In October 1742, following unruly scenes when the doors had been opened to admit a new batch of applicants, a system of balloting was introduced using a bag of red, white and black balls. If a mother drew a white ball, her child would be admitted if healthy; a red ball placed them on a waiting list, and black ball meant outright rejection.

The Foundling Hospital became the capital's most popular charity and was supported by the greatest artists of the time such as Reynolds and Gainsborough who donated paintings. One of its most notable

patrons was William Hogarth, himself a foundling, who had no children of his own. He designed the charity's coat of arms and uniforms
for the Hospital's inmates. He was also appointed as an 'Inspector for
Wet Nurses', and he and his wife Jane fostered a number of foundling children. Another supporter was the composer George Frideric
Handel, who gave benefit performances of his work in the Hospital
chapel and also provided it with an organ. The music in the chapel on
Sundays became a special attraction and the choir, composed of the
children themselves, was assisted at various times by many of the most
distinguished singers of the day. After morning service on Sundays,
visitors were able to observe the children at dinner.

In 1756, as a condition for receiving a substantial parliamentary
grant, the Hospital was required to adopt an open-ended admissions
policy, taking any child presented who was under the age of two
months (later increased to twelve months). A basket was then placed
on the Hospital's gate where a child could be left and a bell rung to
announce its presence to the staff. Perhaps, not surprisingly, the
Hospital was inundated with infants from far and wide, many being
offloaded from parish workhouses. A trade soon grew up among
vagrants who offered, for a fee, to convey an infant to the Hospital.

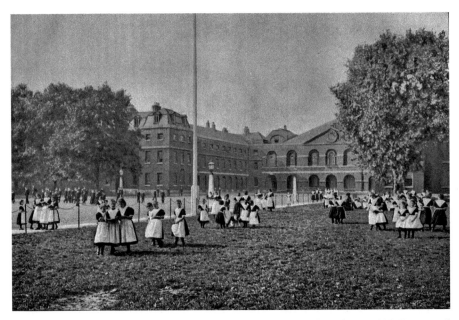

Children at play in front of London's Foundling Hospital in about 1900. Boys and
girls had their own separate areas.

Many such children did not survive their journey or died soon after arrival. Others were just dumped by their courier, who in some cases even removed and sold the child's clothing. The overall mortality rate in this trade was reckoned to be in the order of 70 per cent.[12]

The era of indiscriminate admission ended in 1760 when it was calculated that the cost of the exercise had now risen to around £500,000. Parliamentary support for the scheme was withdrawn and the Hospital was forced to rely on its own funds, charitable support, and payments by parishes for the maintenance of children that they placed. From 1756 to 1801, a procedure also operated where a child could be accepted on payment of £100.

Early London Orphanages

From the second half of the eighteenth century, a growing number of other homes or 'asylums' for orphan children were founded in and around London. These included the Orphan Working School, Hampstead (1758), the Female Orphan Asylum, Lambeth (1758), the St Pancras Female Orphanage (1776), the Home for Female Orphans, St John's Wood (1786) and the London Orphan Asylum, Clapton (1813).

The St Anne's Society (later known as the Royal Asylum of St Anne's Society) might also be included in this group. The Society was founded in 1702 by Thomas Bray, Robert Nelson, and other gentlemen in the parish of St Anne and St Agnes, Aldersgate. The Society's initial object was to clothe and educate twelve sons, orphaned or otherwise, of parents who had been reduced to a necessitous condition. It was only in the 1790s that the Society began to provide residential accommodation on a modest scale, moving in 1829 to large, purpose-built premises in Streatham Hill in South London.

Rather more typical of these early institutions was the Female Orphan Asylum in Lambeth. Its founding, in 1758, was largely through the efforts of Sir John Fielding, who raised donations for an establishment 'to preserve friendless and deserted girls under twelve years of age, from that state of wretchedness which might expose them to all the miseries of prostitution'.[13] The Asylum's original premises were a former inn, called the Hercules' Pillars, at the junction of Westminster Bridge Road and Westminster Road, Southwark, with the first children being admitted in July 1758. The girls were taught and employed in reading, knitting, sewing, making the beds, kitchen work, etc. with the intention of making them 'good housewives, and useful members of society'.[14]

The London Orphan Asylum was founded by the Reverend (later Sir) Andrew Reed, a minister in the Congregational church and a prolific philanthropist. Though not a rich man himself, Reed was particularly effective at raising money for his schemes from wealthy and prestigious donors such as City merchants. During the 1820s, Reed became increasingly concerned about the lack of charitably funded homes for children under 7, the lowest age at which many institutions allowed admission. These included Reed's own London Orphan Asylum, whose rules in this matter its Board of Governors were unwilling to change. He therefore decided to create a new establishment, the Wanstead Infant Orphan Asylum, which he founded in 1827. Reed always believed that philanthropy should be non-denominational and in 1844 set up the Asylum for Fatherless Children in response to the insistence of the governors of his Infant Orphan Asylum that Church of England catechisms be used there. In 1858,

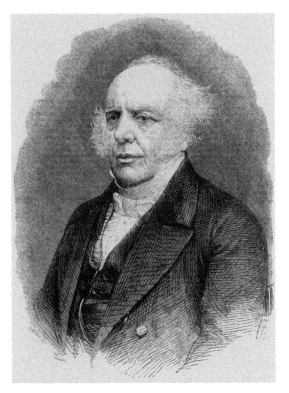

Sir Andrew Reed (1787–1862) who founded the London Orphan Asylum, the Infant Orphan Asylum, the Asylum for Fatherless Children and the Earlswood Asylum for Idiots.

after occupying several temporary premises, the Asylum for Fatherless Children moved to Purley, Surrey, and became known as the Reedham Orphanage.

Many orphanages began life in small rented premises and, if they attracted sufficient support, were late able to move to more spacious, purpose-built accommodation. Sometimes, a further relocation to an even grander building in the countryside might later take place. Typical of this progression was the Female Orphan Asylum whose original premises were rebuilt in 1824 as three sides of a quadrangle. Its chapel was open to the public on Sundays and collections were made for the benefit of the children 'whose cleanly and healthy appearance cannot fail to interest the spectators'.[15] In 1866, the orphanage moved to Beddington, near Croydon, to an ancient mansion house called Carew Manor, where accommodation was provided for 150 girls.

Like all charitable enterprises, fund-raising was always a concern for those running children's homes. Annual subscriptions and one-off donations provided much of their income, and lists of subscribers and donors were invariably featured in the organization's annual report, or even published in local newspapers. Attracting patronage from the nobility could boost both the reputation and, more importantly, the income of a charitable institution, with royal endorsement virtually being a guarantee of successful fund-raising. In 1850, Queen Victoria

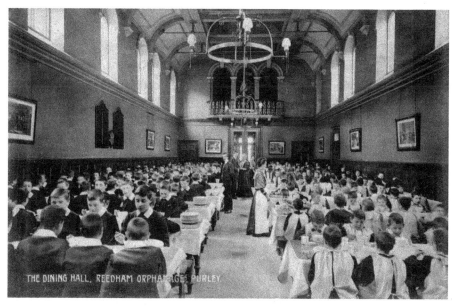

The dining-hall at the Reedham Orphanage, Purley, early 1900s.

TO THE GOVERNORS OF & SUBSCRIBERS TO THE

THE BRITISH ORPHAN ASYLUM.

Your Votes and Interest are most respectfully and earnestly solicited in behalf of

JOHN RUSSELL,

AGED SEVEN YEARS.

FATHER AND MOTHER BOTH DEAD.

The Orphan's Father was formerly a Poulterer in King Street, Westminster. Both Parents, and two Brothers, 11 and 2 years of age, died within five days, last September, from MALIGNANT CHOLERA, at 50, Queen's Row, Walworth; which leaves the Orphan dependent upon his maternal Aunt, who already maintains her own Mother by dress-making.

This Case is earnestly recommended by

Rev. C. WORDSWORTH, D.D., Canon of Westm.	WM. BOUTCHER, Esq., Denmark Hill
Rev. T. W. MELLER, M.A., Woodbridge, Suffolk	Rev. J. JENNINGS, M.A., Canon of Westminster
Rev. F.F. STATHAM, B.A., St. Peter's, Walworth	R. A. GREY, Esq., Camberwell Terrace
Rev. GEO. AINSLIE, M.A., Park St., Westminster	Rev. R. FAYRER, Emanuel Church, Camberwell
Rev. TEMPLE FREERE, M.A., Canon of West-	WM. MORTIMORE, Esq., Champion Hill
minster	Rev. H. HUTTON, M.A., St.Paul's, Covent Garden
Rev. DANIEL MOORE, Camden Church	Rev. J. A.COOK, M.A., St.Margaret's, Westminster

Proxies will be most thankfully received by Miss Meller, Denmark Hill, and the Rev. G. Ainslie, M.A., Park Street, Westminster.

A lobbying card sent to voters electing new entrants at the British Orphan Asylum, pleading the case of 7-year-old orphan John Russell.

became the patron of the Orphan Working School in Hampstead, also making a donation of 250 guineas to the institution. This allowed her to nominate, for the duration of her lifetime, one inmate for the establishment. The first child to receive the royal nomination was named Joseph Parrett, whose mother had died from cholera.

None of these institutions had unlimited places, however, and those they took in often spent their whole childhood there. When spaces did become available, the selection of those to be admitted was usually by a periodic ballot of the charity's subscribers. Applicants were usually required to be orphans, to have been born in wedlock and to be in good physical health. The Orphan Working School refused entry to all children who had ever resided in a prison or workhouse, many of whom would have been illegitimate. When admission ballots were approaching, those who were eligible to vote were often lobbied by the supporters of a particular applicant pleading their case.

Outside London

Although the charity school movement spread across the whole of England, most of the schools limited their activities to educating their pupils and perhaps also supplying meals and clothing. The number providing residential accommodation was always fairly modest, perhaps fewer than fifty, with an average of thirty or so places in each.[16] The gradual appearance of children's 'asylums' and orphanages that took place in London in the eighteenth century was not replicated elsewhere, however. In the rest of the country, it was the poor-relief authorities that were effectively at the forefront in providing residential care for orphan and destitute children in the form of the workhouse – another institution much promoted by the SPCK.

In 1698, in Kingston upon Hull, the town's recently formed Corporation of the Poor erected a large new workhouse known as Charity Hall. Originally intended to house the poor of all ages, it was instead used for many years as a home and training school for the town's orphan and destitute children.

At Bristol, also in 1698, the Corporation of the Poor rented a building for use as a workhouse to house a hundred pauper girls. The girls were taught reading and the older ones carried out all the housework of the establishment. They also learned to spin and were hired out to local manufacturers. However, the coarseness of the yarn they produced soon resulted in complaints and low payment rates. The following year, the Corporation purchased a house that had recently been occupied by the Treasury as a mint and so became known as the Mint Workhouse. It was used to house the elderly, young children, and a hundred boys. The boys were occupied in spinning cotton wool and weaving fustian, for which they were able to generate the creditable income of £6 per week. The boys were also taught to read and, unlike the girls, to write.

A similar pattern was followed to a greater or lesser degree in many of the hundreds of parish workhouses that were set up during the eighteenth century. In these establishments, the children among the inmates would typically be educated for a few hours each day, usually in the morning, then work for the rest of the time, either in domestic chores or in some textile-related activity such as spinning, weaving, combing or sewing. Apart from producing clothing for themselves or other workhouse inmates, or even generating a cash income, the children's labour could provide them with useful skills for adult life. In many cases, employment or apprenticeship would be arranged for them on leaving the workhouse. The hope – not always fulfilled – was that they would then never again need to be supported by the parish.

Chapter 2

Reformatories, Ragged and Industrial Schools

Reformatories

Attempts to provide care for children involved in criminal or anti-social behaviour – often referred to as 'juvenile delinquents' – date back to at least the eighteenth century. An early initiative began in 1756 with the founding of the Marine Society 'for the purpose of clothing landsmen and boys for the use of the king's ship, and as an expedient to provide for poor boys who might become a nuisance'.[1] The Society was a pioneer in the use of training ships for this work (see chapter 4).

In 1788, the Philanthropic Society was set up 'for the protection of poor children, and the offsprings of convicted felons; and for the reformation of those who have themselves been engaged in criminal practices'.[2] In the same year, the Society opened an institution at St George's Fields, Southwark, whose facilities included male and female 'Reforms'. The inmates manufactured items such as clothes, shoes and rope, and were given religious instruction.

In the first part of the nineteenth century, penalties for those found guilty of crimes would, by modern standards, be considered exceptionally severe. In 1833, a boy of 9 was sentenced to death (though not actually executed) for stealing 2d. worth of paint.[3] Two boys of 15 were transported for seven years for stealing a pair of boots. Such treatment began to be questioned and in 1837 Parkhurst prison, on the Isle of Wight, was used to provide an experimental reformatory regime for young offenders. They were provided with outdoor industrial training, combined with school instruction and religious teaching. The establishment had mixed results and was eventually closed, with the authorities indicating that private or charitably run establishments were preferable for such purposes.

Scotland made an important contribution to the development of Reformatories with the opening of the Glasgow Boys' House of Refuge

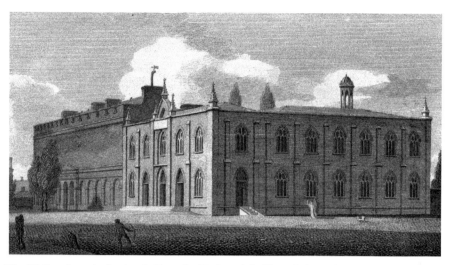

The Philanthropic Society's Female 'Reform' (left) and chapel at St George's in the Fields, in about 1805.

in 1838 and the city's House of Refuge for Females two years later. Both offered young offenders an alternative to prison with a regime of education and vocational training.

In 1846, Lord Houghton attempted to introduce a Parliamentary Bill to establish a national system of Reformatory Schools as an alternative to prison for convicted juvenile offenders. Although the Bill did not become law, it led to growing interest in such a scheme, with the Philanthropic Society again at the forefront of the movement. In 1849, members of the Society visited the agricultural colony for delinquent boys in Mettray in France, where the inmates lived in family-style groups. The Society subsequently established a pioneering farm colony for boys in Redhill in Surrey, based on the Mettray model.

A leading figure in the Reformatory School movement was Mary Carpenter, author of the influential 1851 book *Reformatory Schools for the Children of the Perishing and Dangerous Classes, and for Juvenile Offenders*. Much influenced by the regime adopted at Mettray, Carpenter believed that the treatment of Reformatory inmates should be based on the love of the child and, ideally, provide a family-sized environment. She also considered that there should be no forced work, that recreation and sport should be provided and that corporal punishment be kept to a minimum. Another prominent supporter of the Reformatory movement was Matthew Davenport Hill. In his post as the Recorder of

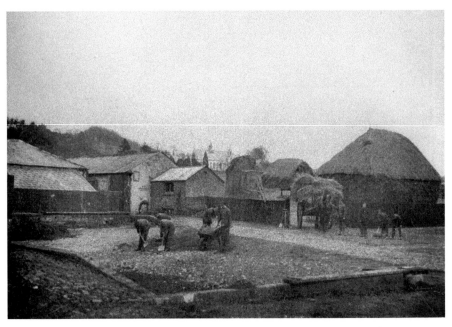

Boys at work in the rickyard at the Philanthropic Society's boys' reformatory in Redhill.

Birmingham, where he sat as a judge in court proceedings, he refused to send children to prison.

In 1851, the first conference on Preventive and Reformatory Schools was held in Birmingham, following which several new voluntary institutions were established by individuals who were keen to put their ideas into practice. These included:

- Kingswood Reformatory, near Bristol, opened in 1852 by Mary Carpenter and Russell Scott.
- Saltley Reformatory, near Birmingham, founded in 1852 by Charles Adderley, MP.
- Stoke Farm Reformatory, Worcestershire, established in 1853 by Joseph Sturge.
- Red Lodge Reformatory, Bristol, opened in 1854 by Mary Carpenter.

Mary Carpenter's writings and her evidence to an 1852 parliamentary inquiry on juvenile delinquents helped shape the Youthful Offenders Act of 1854. The Act enabled voluntary bodies to operate reformatories which would be formally certified as 'useful and efficient' by the

Inspector of Prisons and subjected to regular inspection. Convicted juvenile offenders, under the age of 16, could be granted a pardon on condition that they were committed to a Certified Reformatory School for a period of two to five years. Those entering Reformatories were first required to spend a period of fourteen days in prison. Parents of inmates were required to contribute to the cost of their child's maintenance by a payment to the institution of up to five shillings a week, with the government making up any shortfall.

The initial prison requirement imposed on those placed in reformatories was viewed by many as counter-productive and was campaigned against by a group of magistrates, MPs, and social reformers such as Mary Carpenter. After this proved unsuccessful, they proposed the creation of an alternative institution, the Certified Industrial School, aimed at a younger age group and without the prison element. The suggestion was taken up and eventually put into law, first by the Reformatory Schools (Scotland) Act of 1854 (also known as Dunlop's Act) which, despite its title, was solely concerned with under-14s found begging or wandering. The same idea was also the focus of the Industrial Schools Act of 1857, which applied to England and Wales.

Ragged and Industrial Schools

Industrial Schools were not a new idea, but had their roots in the Ragged School movement which had developed over the previous half-century. Ragged schools were aimed at the poorest children – those who were invariably dressed in rags – who could not gain admission to any existing institutions. Charles Dickens commented that 'Sunday and Day Schools of the humblest class were "too respectable" apparently for these youngsters, who had a raggedness and dirtiness which defied classification, and demanded an establishment of their own.'[4] The Schools provided free lessons and, in many cases, meals to those who attended. Instruction in practical skills, often referred to as 'industrial' training, also came to be a common feature of the Schools.

A pioneer in the development of ragged schools was Thomas Cranfield, a tailor and former soldier, who between 1798 and his death in 1838, built up a network of Sunday night and infants' schools situated in the poorest parts of London.

Another significant figure was the Portsmouth shoemaker, John Pounds, who, following an accident in his teens, became known as the 'crippled cobbler'. In 1818, when in his fifties, Pounds began giving local poor children free lessons in reading, writing, arithmetic, Bible study, carpentry, shoemaking and cookery.

Scotland played an important part in the development of ragged schools. In 1841, in response to learning that hundreds of Aberdeen's children were common beggars and thieves, the city's Sheriff, William Watson, established a ragged school for boys. The pupils were taught reading and writing, and worked at teasing hair and making salmon nets. They received breakfast, dinner and supper at the school and were forbidden to beg. Despite some initial local opposition to the scheme, it proved a success and an establishment for girls followed two years later. On 9 May 1845, Watson launched his 'Soup Kitchen' school, to which the city's police agreed to bring every child they found begging. Over the day, seventy-five were collected, of whom only four could read. The proceedings were far from peaceful: 'Confusion and uproar, quarrelling and fighting, language of the most hateful description, and the most determined rebellion against everything like order and regularity, gave the gentlemen engaged in the undertaking of taming them the hardest day's work they have ever encountered in their lives.'[5]

In Edinburgh, the Reverend Thomas Guthrie promoted Watson's work through his 1847 pamphlet *A Plea for Ragged Schools; or, Prevention Better than Cure*. In the same year, Guthrie set up three schools in Edinburgh, at which children received food, education and industrial training.

In 1844, the Ragged School Union was founded in London, with Lord Ashley (later known as the Earl of Shaftesbury) as its President. The Union eventually had a membership of around 200 establishments. These included Schools not only in the capital, but across the country, mostly in the larger towns and cities. Reflecting their training provision, many of the Schools began to include the word 'industrial' in their name.

Bristol's first ragged school, 'for the instruction and moral improvement of those whose poverty, habits and mode of procuring subsistence, have unfitted them for belonging to any other school', was founded by Mary Carpenter, with the support of local surgeon John Bishop Estlin. The School was opened in August 1846 in a room in Lewin's Mead and Mr Grant engaged as master. Operations were begun by the master's going out into Lewin's Mead, a street 'notorious for the general vicious character of its population', and collecting around him a number of the idle and lawless boys who abounded in the district, and telling them he was going to open a school the following day, which would be free to anyone who would come to learn how to read and write.[6] Some immediately agreed to come, while others wanted to know what the master would give them if they attended. They were told that he had nothing to give them 'but such instruction as would enable them to instruct themselves, and to become useful, honest, and happy boys'. At nine o'clock the next morning, three boys presented themselves at the school room, and in the afternoon thirteen or fourteen came. The new arrivals were far from placid, however. According to the master, there was 'some swearing, some fighting, some crying. One boy struck another's head through the window. I tried to offer up a short prayer, but found it impossible: the boys, instead of kneeling, began to tumble over one another, and to sing *Jim Crow*.'[7]

The master persisted and, within a few weeks, there was a regular attendance of thirty boys, varying in age from 6 or 7 up to 17 years. It was then decided to move the school to larger premises and to open it in the evenings. The hours at the new school were, on weekdays, 10 to 12, 2 to 4 and 7 to 9, except for Saturday afternoon and evening. On Sunday, the hours were 9 to 11 in the morning and 6 to 8 in the evening. Instruction was given in reading, writing and arithmetic, with other subjects judged conducive to intellectual, moral, and religious improvement. No payment was required of the pupils. The school was open to the poor of every religious creed, or of no creed at all, and the

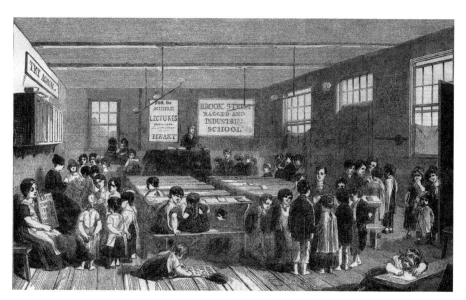

A classroom at the Brook Street Ragged and Industrial School, 1853.

instruction was entirely non-sectarian. At first, the school was for boys only, but girls were later admitted.

At some ragged schools, a limited amount of residential accommodation began to be provided for homeless and destitute children. Sunderland's Industrial and Ragged Schools – the plural indicating separate sections for boys and girls – opened their doors in 1850, and by November 1851 had sixty children in residence. The Birmingham Free Industrial School moved to new premises in 1850 which provided a day school, industrial classes and a residential 'asylum' for deserted and orphan children.

Shoeblack Brigades

On 28 November 1850, a group of ragged school teachers met to consider potential ways in which the boys they taught might be able to gain new employment when the Great Exhibition took place the following summer. After the meeting, three of the attendees, R. J. Shape, John MacGregor and J. R. Fowler, were walking along Holborn together when one of them made the suggestion that some of the boys work as shoeblacks, cleaning the shoes and boots of foreign visitors, as happened in Paris. The three pledged money for the idea and began to promote the scheme, raise funds and form a committee.

At a public meeting on 19 January 1851, at the Field Lane Ragged School, a demonstration was given by the first recruit to the Shoeblack Brigade. A young man, a former expert thief, mounted the platform in his uniform of a bright red jersey and black apron, and equipped with a blacking-box, foot-stand and brushes, showed how the work would be done. The Honorary Secretary said the arrangement envisaged locating a number of boys at various points on metropolitan thoroughfares, to provide to visitors, throughout the summer, clean shoes, with civility and at a standard charge of one penny. It was reported that several kind ladies had provided thirty uniforms, ten boxes and five sets of brushes, and that an inspector would shortly be appointed. On 24 February, a training base was set up in some rented rooms near John Street, in the Strand. At the end of March, five boys began work, the first in a corner of Leicester Square. An observer of the occasion recorded that:

Oh! I was very anxious to see whether anybody would employ the shoe-black; and glad indeed was I to observe a good, honest, fat-sided Englishman approach the little boy and place his great boot upon the top of his box. The boy touched his cap, set to work upon his knees, smartly brushed the mud from the man's trousers, turned them carefully up, attacked the muddy leather with vigour, and soon made it a yellow-grey, then he applied the blacking and briskly plied the polisher until the boot was bright. So was the other foot finished. The man paid his penny, the boy touched his cap, and the work was done. Another, and another, and another, came and paid and went. First, a clerk wishing to show off at his office, then a milliner girl who had spattered her thin shoes, next a burly farmer striding along in his huge top boots, a fish-wife next, a whiskered foreigner, and then a peer of the realm. The shoe-blacks that day obtained a footing in London.[8]

Pitches were allocated to the boys by the police, with the Brigade operating along the Strand, Piccadilly, Regent Street, Holborn and in the Parks. Because some locations were more lucrative than others, the allocation of pitches was changed twice a week.

In 1851, the year of the Great Exhibition, a team of thirty-seven boys cleaned 165,000 pairs of shoes, producing an income of £650.[9] After the Exhibition closed in October, five of the boys immigrated to America.

Following the example of what became known as the Central or 'Reds' Shoeblack Brigade, the movement gradually spread across the whole of London, with around a dozen Brigades eventually being formed, each with its own distinctive uniform. Some Brigades made a point of including boys with various forms of disability such as the deaf and dumb and the physically disabled – what were then usually referred to as 'cripples'. In most cases, the Brigades also provided hostel-style accommodation for their members.

In the Central and most other Brigades, the boys' earnings were paid into the home each day with a third of the money paying for their keep, a third being placed into their individual bank savings accounts, and a third given back to them. To encourage honesty and application, prizes ranging from 3s. 6d. down to 6d. were awarded each month. The West London Brigade adopted an alternative system where the boys paid 1s. 6d. a week for lodging and for their board according to what they consumed. They also paid from 4d. to 1s. 8d. a day for their pitches, according to the location.

The Shoeblack Brigades had largely disappeared by the onset of the First World War. Shoe-shining continued as a London street trade for many years, however, although by the 1960s it had virtually vanished. Boys' Shoeblack Brigades were also started in a number of other towns such as Brighton, Liverpool, Leeds, Manchester and Dublin.

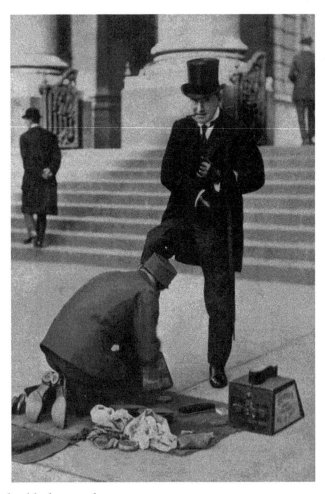

A London shoeblack at work.

Certified Industrial Schools

The establishments specified in the 1857 Industrial Schools Act became known as Certified Industrial Schools. Children aged from 7 to 14 who had been convicted of vagrancy could be placed in a Certified Industrial School until they reached the age of 16, regardless of their age of entry. A further Industrial Schools Act in 1861 defined four categories of potential entrants: under-14s found begging, under-14s found wandering and homeless or frequenting with thieves, under-12s who had committed an imprisonable offence and under-14s who parents could not control them. Parents of an offender committed to an Industrial School could be ordered to pay up to three shillings a week (increased to five shillings in 1861) towards their child's maintenance.

Like Reformatories, the Schools required official accreditation as to the suitability of their premises, facilities, staffing and management before they received children placed by the courts. Thereafter, they received official inspections on a regular basis, usually two or three times a year.

In June 1858, the first two Industrial Schools to be certified under the new system were the Tre-wint Industrial School in Hackney and the York Ragged and Industrial Schools, both establishments that had already been in operation for a number of years. Others soon followed in Manchester, Liverpool, Newcastle, Bristol and Coventry, although London accounted for half of the first twenty institutions to be accredited.

Industrial Schools that had previously operated as ragged schools sometimes continued in a dual role with local children attending classes on a daily basis alongside inmates who were under confinement. Those that converted from ragged schools were often mixed establishments, while newly founded ones were usually single-sex institutions. Since the number of girls committed by the courts was always much lower than the number of boys, the Home Office

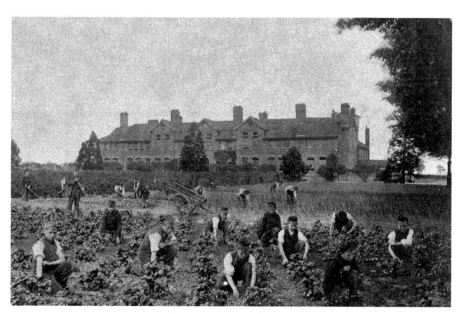

Essex Industrial School for Boys, Chelmsford, early 1900s – the inmates are occupied in agricultural work.

viewed single-sex establishments as more efficient in their use of staff resources and premises, and as providing a better environment for the girls. Between 1875 and 1905, largely as a result of official pressure, the number of mixed Industrial Schools in England fell from thirteen to two.[10] Reformatories were all single-sex, with the brief exception of Mary Carpenter's establishment in Kingswood.

Many Industrial Schools received voluntary admissions as well as those committed by the courts. The attraction of gaining Industrial School certification, however, was the income it brought for each inmate's maintenance. This was something of particular benefit to establishments that struggled to get by on charitable donations, even if parents sometimes had to be chased for their weekly payments. There was no guarantee, however, that local magistrates would commit offenders to any particular Industrial School and some soon closed due to their lack of uptake.

After spending at least eighteen months in an Industrial School, inmates could be released on a rolling three-month licence to live with a 'trustworthy and respectable person'. If they escaped from the person with whom they were placed under licence, or refused to return to the School on the revocation or expiry of their licence, they were deemed to have escaped from the School and would be dealt with accordingly. This might result in transfer to a Reformatory.

Further Legislation

In 1860, central supervision of Industrial Schools passed from the Committee of Council on Education into the hands of the Home Office.

The Industrial Schools Act of 1866 widened the categories of eligible children to include destitute children whose parents were in prison, and children in the care of the workhouse authorities whose behaviour was deemed to be 'refractory'. The Act also transferred overall responsibility for both Reformatory and Industrial Schools to the Inspectors of Prisons, with a single inspector covering both types of establishment.

Following the 1869 Habitual Criminals Act, children under 14 of women twice convicted of 'crime' could be sent to an Industrial School. From 1880, this was extended to under-14s found to be living in a brothel, or living with or associating with common or reputed prostitutes.

In 1899, the initial prison requirement for those entering a Reformatory was abolished. This reduced the difference between

Reformatory Schools and Certified Industrial Schools, although the latter broadly dealt with a younger age group and included those who were deemed to be in danger of becoming criminals rather than necessarily having committed offences.

Life in Reformatory and Industrial Schools

Although the inmates of Reformatory and Industrial Schools differed in their reasons for being there, and the age ranges received at the two institutions were not the same, the strictly regimented regime that was implemented for the inmates was largely similar.

Classroom education at the Schools included the basics of reading, writing and arithmetic (or ciphering, as it was sometimes known). Mental arithmetic received much attention as it was not only a useful skill but could be quickly tested by an inspector. Other lessons frequently included recitation, composition, history, geography and, by the 1890s, drawing. Singing and the rudiments of music were also widely taught.

Outside the classroom, industrial training formed an important part of the daily routine. In both boys' and girls' Schools, the inmates were expected to perform a significant part, or even all, of the domestic labour of the institution. This included working in the kitchen and laundry, and general household tasks such as making and changing beds and cleaning. In institutions that drew their water from a well, for example the Standon Farm School, the inmates could be employed in operating the water pumps. Chopping firewood was another task that – in boys' Schools at least – was often undertaken, with some of the production generating an income through its sale to local householders. In 1892, it was reckoned that the wood-chopping machine at York Industrial School could turn out 8,000 bundles of firewood a day.[11]

As far as vocational training was concerned, the girls were invariably prepared for future employment as domestic servants. Apart from their on-the-job experience doing the household chores, they were usually taught needlework, knitting and dressmaking, and sometimes made their own clothing. Some Schools later introduced lessons in subjects such as cookery and domestic economy. At Leeds, as well as making their own outfits, the inmates of the Girls' Industrial School made all the socks and shirts for the nearby Boys' Reformatory.[12]

The boys often had a much more varied range of opportunities on offer, with training in trades such as carpentry, blacksmithing, brush-making, basket-making, tailoring, shoemaking and clog-making. As with the girls, the various trades could often supply much of the School's

	WEEKDAYS		SUNDAYS
A.M.		A.M.	
5.30–6.00	Rise, Dress, Private Prayers, Wash, etc.	7.00–8.00	Rise, Dress, Private Prayers, Wash, etc.
6.00–7.45	Schooling, Winter months. In Summer, out to Work.	8.00–9.00	Breakfast, Family Prayers, &c.
7.45–8.45	Family Prayers, read Psalms for the day, and Breakfast	9.00–10.00	Religious Instruction
8.45–1.00	Industrial Employment. On wet days, schooling.	10.00–1.00	Church
P.M.		P.M.	
1.00–2.00	Assemble. Wash, Dinner, Recreation	1.00–2.30	Dinner and Recreation
2.00–5.30	Industrial Employment	2.30–4.30	Religious Instruction. Collects and Gospel, or Church in Winter
5.30–6.30	Assemble, Wash, Supper	4.30–5.30	Supper and Recreation
6.30–8.30	Schooling	5.30–6.00	Prepare for Church
8.30–8.45	Family Prayers, Private Prayers, and bed	6.00–8.00	Church or Religious Instruction, Singing Hymns, Reading, &c., and bed
*	Stock boys, Cooks, Tailors, rise at 5.30 a.m. in charge of Officer, and changed alternately.		Stock boys rise at 6 a.m., with Officer in Charge, also Cook and Post Boy.

NOTE:–On Saturdays, the boys cease work out of doors at 1.30 p.m. Saturday afternoons and evenings are spent in preparing for Sunday – bathing, changing linen, recreation, Scripture, and learning Collects and Gospels, &c., &c.

Every inmate is bathed once a fortnight, and during the summer months the boys are allowed to bathe once or twice in the Canal, and learn to swim.

August, 1870. (Signed) THOMAS GEE, Governor.

Daily timetable in 1870 at the Hardwicke Boys' Reformatory, Gloucestershire.[13]

	BREAKFAST	DINNER	SUPPER
Sunday	1 pint Boiled Milk and Bread, with Coffee, or Oatmeal Porridge occasionally. Bread ad libitum.	3 & 4 oz. Cooked Meat, with Potatoes. Bread ad libitum.	1 pint of Tea. Bread ad libitum.
Monday	"	Potato Hash, made with Meat. Bread ad libitum.	1 pint Boiled Milk and Bread, or Oatmeal Porridge or Coffee. Bread ad libitum.
Tuesday	"	2½ & 3 oz. Cooked Meat, Potatoes. Bread ad libitum.	"
Wednesday	"	Potato Pie, or Hash, made with Meat.	"
Thursday	"	Bacon (2½ & 3 oz.) and Cabbage. Bread ad libitum.	"
Friday	"	Bread Puddings, & 1½ oz. Cheese. Bread ad libitum.	"
Saturday	"	Meat Soup, made with Peas, Rice, or Pearl Barley, and Vegetables. Bread ad libitum.	"

The 'plain and wholesome' diet at Mount St Bernard's Boys' Reformatory, 1866.[14]

own requirements from its workshops. In the 1890s, at the Cannington Industrial School for Roman Catholic Boys in Somerset, all the clothes, boots and socks were made by the inmates, while the carpenters contributed to the maintenance of the building. Some Schools had their own bakehouse where the boys learned bread-making and also supplied the institution's daily requirements. A few of the boys' establishments, such as Liverpool's Holy Trinity Industrial School, set up printing departments which, as well as being a training resource, could generate useful income from the outside work they undertook. Boys' Schools in rural

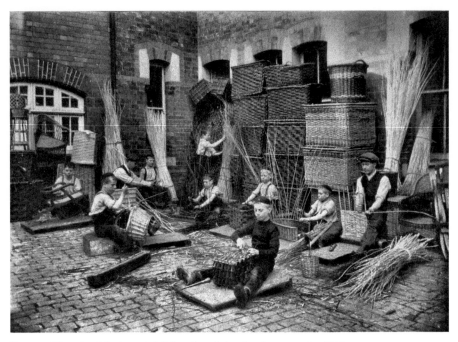

Boys at Hereford Industrial School making baskets, early 1900s.

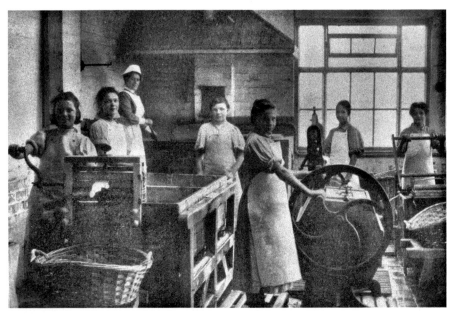

Girls in the laundry at the Coventry Industrial School, about 1910.

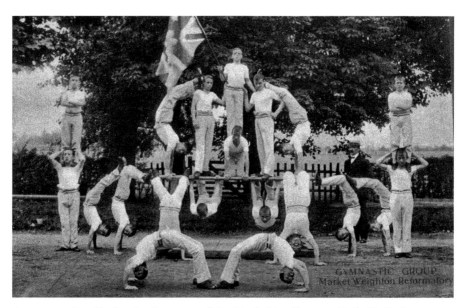

A gymnastics display by inmates of the Yorkshire Roman Catholic Reformatory for Boys in Market Weighton, Yorkshire, early 1900s.

areas, sometimes referred to as Farm Schools, often made a speciality of agricultural training and bought or rented large areas of land for the inmates to cultivate. In 1896, for example, the farmland at the Buxton Reformatory in Norfolk extended to more than fifty acres and had a considerable amount of stock, including pigs and poultry. Market gardens were also established at some institutions that often sold their fruit and vegetables in the local area. For many years, the Standon Industrial School had a stall for their produce at the Stoke-on-Trent market.[15]

The 'training' provided at some institutions, particularly for the younger inmates at Industrial Schools, could be rather limited, with menial tasks such as hair teasing, oakum picking and matchbox or paperbag-making being employed.

Exercise and sport were always considered an important part of a School's regime, particularly for boys, with a good-sized playground and playing field being rated as important by inspectors. Games such as football and cricket were popular, with some schools' teams being regularly successful in local leagues. Swimming was also encouraged, with many Schools installing a swimming bath of some sort. In the 1890s, gymnastics and military-style drill came into vogue. Army sergeant-majors were often employed to put both boys and girls through their paces, with the rather gentler system of Swedish drill sometimes

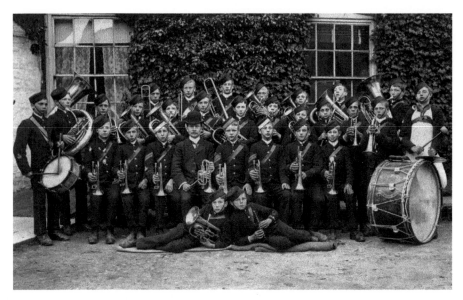

The boys' band at Castle Howard Reformatory, North Yorkshire.

being adopted for the girls. In boys' establishments, a School band was often set up. As well as the band's educational and recreational value, proficiency with a musical instrument could often lead to a future career as a military bandsman. School bands frequently performed at fêtes and other social events in their locality.

Religious education and attendance at services featured prominently in the Schools' routine, with both 'Family' and private prayers at the beginning and end of each day. On Sundays, public worship at some convenient church or chapel was usually arranged. At Anglican institutions, arrangements were required to be made for access to non-Anglican inmates by a minister of the relevant faith.

Visits to inmates by friends or near relatives were generally allowed every two or three months.

Discipline

Discipline at Reformatory and Industrial Schools was strict. At many boys' institutions, corporal punishment, or 'personal chastisement' as it was officially known, was administered frequently. For very serious offences, such as absconding, the official Industrial School regulations decreed that 'whipping shall be inflicted – on the posterior with a birch rod, such punishment not to exceed twelve strokes'. For lesser misdemeanours, up to six strokes could be applied to the palm of the hand with a 'common school cane'.[16] Persistent offenders could be put before magistrates. In the case of Industrial School inmates, this might result in a transfer to a Reformatory, while repeated misconduct by Reformatory inmates could earn them a three-month prison sentence.

In principle, girls were not allowed to be beaten although such punishments could occasionally be sanctioned. Following a mutiny at the Warwickshire Reformatory for Girls in 1923, government inspector Dr A. W. Norris advised the School's superintendent to inflict corporal punishment on the ringleader, 15-year-old Dora Help, which she did forthwith.[17]

The officially sanctioned alternatives to corporal punishment were a loss of rewards and privileges, a reduction in the quality or quantity of food, or confinement in a lighted room or cell. The linking of rewards and privileges to good behaviour was regularly recommended by school inspectors and many institutions introduced mark systems where a weekly or monthly tally of marks or points was required in order to receive visitors or to participate in such activities as sports fixtures. In some cases, small monetary rewards could also be earned by good conduct. Part of the money might be held back and put into a savings account and released to the individual in stages after they left the School.

Licence and Discharge

After eighteen months in a Reformatory or Industrial School, an inmate could be released on licence to live with a specified 'trustworthy and respectable person'. So long as no further misconduct occurred, the licence could be repeatedly renewed for three months at a time until the end of the detention period. Refusing to return to the School at the end of a licence period, or escaping from the allocated person, was treated as absconding from the School and punished accordingly.

The decision to license out any particular inmate was at the discretion of the School's superintendent. There was, however, often some reluctance to license out inmates. Schools liked to keep their occupancy rates reasonably high. Apart from financial considerations, any reduction in the number of inmates could reduce the workforce available to run the institution, with the inmates who had been there the longest often making the most significant contribution to the labour force.

At the end of their detention period or, in the case of an Industrial School, on reaching the age of 16, inmates were provided with an outfit of clothing and, where practicable, placed in employment or service. From 1891, apprenticeship or emigration could be arranged prior to the normal discharge date.

Day Industrial Schools

The 1870 Education Act was the first statute to deal specifically with the provision of education in Britain. Among its most significant measures, the Act enabled the formation of local School Boards in areas where existing educational provision was inadequate.

A subsequent Education Act in 1876 allowed School Boards to establish Industrial Schools and also a new type of institution – Day Industrial Feeding Schools. The latter, usually referred to just as Day Industrial Schools, arose from a proposal in 1873 by the Bristol School Board. They suggested that there was a useful role for an institution that provided remedial care and training for children for those failing to attend ordinary Board Schools but that did not entirely remove them from ordinary family life. In the 1876 Act, Day Industrial Schools were specified as being 'for those children whose education is neglected by their parents, or who are found wandering or in bad company'. The Schools were defined as institutions 'in which industrial training, elementary education, and one or more meals a day, but not lodging, are provided for the children' for their 'proper training and control'. Children typically attended the Schools between 8 a.m. and 6 p.m. and received all their meals there. Satisfactory attendance at a School would allow a child, on licence, to return to an ordinary school.

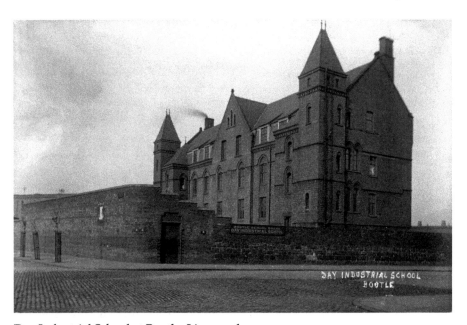

Day Industrial School at Bootle, Liverpool.

Day Industrial Schools were established almost immediately by School Boards in Bristol and Liverpool, soon followed by Gateshead, Oxford, Yarmouth, and a second school in Liverpool.

Truant Schools

Another new type of Industrial School that appeared following the 1876 Education Act was the Truant School, again operated by local School Boards. This was an institution to which magistrates could commit children up to the age of 14 who persistently refused to attend elementary schools.

Truant Schools provided a strict regime with, for example, play-time replaced by marching drill. After a period of typically one to three months, the offender was released on a renewable licence to attend an ordinary elementary school. Any further truancy resulted in the child's being returned to the Truant School to be faced with corporal punishment and a lengthier period of confinement before being re-released on licence. The first Truant Schools to be established, in 1878, were

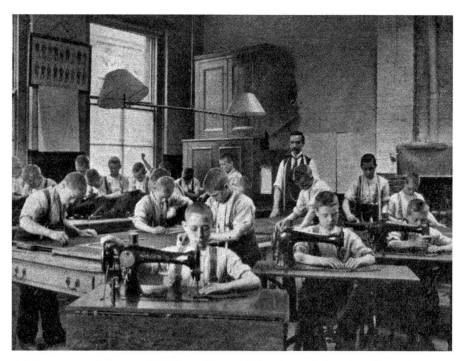

A tailoring workshop at Highbury Truant School, north London. Some boys are cutting out cloth, others sewing by hand or by machine.

in London and Liverpool, with around sixteen eventually in operation. From 1908, Truant Industrial Schools were renamed Short-Term Industrial Schools.

Founders and Managers of Reformatory and Industrial Schools

By 1879, twenty-five years after the 1854 Youthful Offenders Act, there were fifty-two Reformatory Schools in England and Wales, together with ninety-five Industrial Schools. At the same date, Scotland had twelve Reformatory Schools and thirty-four Industrial Schools. A total of seven Day Industrial Schools had then been opened, including one in Scotland, together with three Truant Schools, all of which were in England.

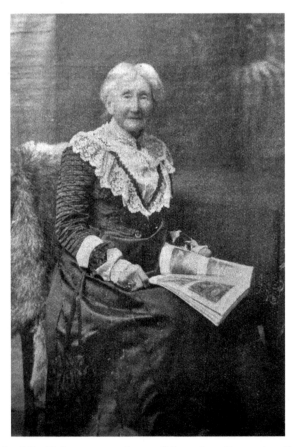

A 1906 portrait of the Reformatory pioneer Mary Ann Carpenter, then aged 98.

A wide variety of groups and individuals were involved in setting up these institutions. In most cases, individual founders became involved in the running of the establishments, either alone or, as more usually happened, with a management committee being formed. The founders and managers broadly fell into four categories: individuals, groups of local magistrates, religious bodies and School Boards.

The efforts of energetic and dedicated individuals provided the driving force behind the creation and operation of many Reformatory and Industrial Schools. The work of Mary Carpenter has already been referred to. The Reformatory she co-founded in 1852 at Kingswood, near Bristol, was initially a mixed establishment, but problems with the behaviour of the female inmates led her to open the Red Lodge Reformatory in Bristol, the first such institution for girls, which she personally superintended from her own residence nearby. The purchase of the Red Lodge premises was financed by Lady Noel Byron, widow of the eminent poet, who shared Carpenter's views on the subject of juvenile reform.

Typical of the less well-known contributors to this work was Joseph Brittain Pash, the head of an agricultural engineering company in Chelmsford, who founded the Essex Industrial School and Home for Destitute Boys in 1872. The School began life in a pair of ordinary houses but in 1879 moved into large, purpose-built premises housing 150 boys. Pash then became the School's resident manager and director, a role he continued until his retirement in 1903.

Institutions run by independent individuals had considerable autonomy. Where there was a formal management committee, it often consisted of friends or relatives invited to serve by the founder. Such committees were not always very active, however. This gradually changed over the years, with moves being made for a School's government funding or certification to be dependent on the proper constitution and operation of its management committee.

Not surprisingly, groups of local magistrates took considerable interest in the emergence of the new institutions that would be available to them when dealing with the fate of young offenders. In 1853, Edmund Antrobus, a Middlesex Justice of the Peace, proposed the founding of a reformatory-style establishment for young offenders in the county. The idea received sufficient support from his fellow magistrates for the passing of special legislation in the form of the 1854 Middlesex Act, pre-empting the Youthful Offenders Act of the same year. However, the resulting institution, the Feltham Industrial School, was on such a grand scale – a Palladian building accommodating up to 800 boys, with two swimming baths among its facilities – that it was not completed until 1859.

On a more modest scale was the Kent County Industrial School for Girls set up by a committee of county magistrates in 1873, in a house in Greenwich. In 1875, the same body opened a rather larger boys' establishment in Kingsnorth, near Ashford. It was named Stanhope School after Lord Stanhope, the committee's chairman, a position he maintained for many years. Managers of magistrate-operated schools were elected and more subject to change than those founded by individuals.

Around a third of Reformatory and Industrial Schools were established and operated by religious groups, with the majority of these being Roman Catholic organizations. Catholic institutions were usually run by religious orders such as the Sisters of Nazareth or the Daughters of Charity of St Vincent de Paul. In such cases, the local Catholic Diocese would, nominally at least, have some involvement in the management of institutions in their area.

Although the Methodist, Jewish and Quaker communities each ran at least one Industrial School, the Church of England's Waifs and Strays Society was the main non-Catholic organization to become involved in their operation. It eventually established seven Industrial Schools including those at Standon Bridge, Hemel Hempstead and Mumbles, near Cardiff. The Society's Schools were managed by local committees in which the local clergy were invariably involved.

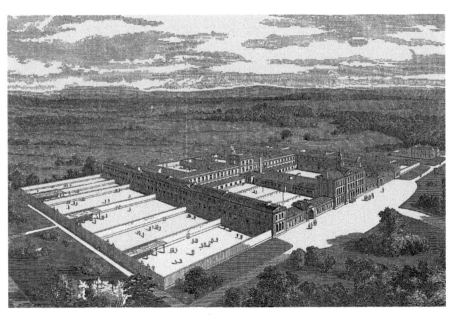

Architect's bird's-eye-view design for the Middlesex Boys' Industrial School, Feltham.

Problems

Those who managed Reformatory and Industrial Schools had to cope with a multitude of potential problems. The numbers of inmates in their institutions and the financial impact of being under-occupied were a frequent concern, as was the cost of maintaining or improving the premises. A high staff turnover, which was often the case with teaching posts, could leave the inmates unsettled, disruptive or even mutinous. By their very nature, those who were committed to a Reformatory or Industrial School were likely to have come from a rough background. In some instances, it was the managers' own inexperience or incompetence that led to problems.

In 1867, some inmates of the Training Refuge for Destitute Girls, at Marylebone, made an unsuccessful attempt to set fire to the premises. The girls themselves immediately raised the alarm and the fire was easily extinguished. The facts about the incident only came to light about two months after the event, when a discharged inmate provided the information. As a result, the managers of the Refuge resolved to resign their Industrial Schools certificate and to continue with only voluntary inmates. The Refuge's inspector thought its managers were overreacting and that reducing its numbers would be detrimental to its future, but was forced to accept their decision.

Much more serious was the twenty-year catalogue of events that took place at the Mount St Bernard's Reformatory, near Whitwick, Leicestershire, in the 1860s and '70s. The School, for Roman Catholic boys, had been opened by an order of Cistercian monks in 1856. An official inspection in November 1859 recorded that the establishment had encountered 'very serious difficulties … arising mainly from the misconduct and inefficiency of the "Brothers"'.[18] In April 1863, a mutiny took place among the inmates. The police were called in and, after a pitched battle, five of the ringleaders were arrested.

In March 1870 a boy named Patrick Lawley used a pair of scissors to stab another inmate, Francis McEwan, after the two had quarrelled. McEwan died a few days later.

In November 1875, another mutiny took place with 160 out the 200 or so inmates escaping. All were soon recaptured and awarded various degrees of punishment, the majority being soundly birched. During a further mutiny in July 1878, around sixty boys escaped after attacking their guards with knives and stealing the keys of the building.

Despite efforts to improve discipline, the School's straggling and disconnected buildings made supervision of the boys difficult. The

School's 1880 inspection report suggested that the School should be entirely re-organized. The estimated £4,000 cost of rebuilding the premises was something that the Abbey was not able to countenance and in July 1881, the School's certificate was withdrawn.

The 1908 Children and Young Persons Act

The 1908 Children and Young Persons Act, sometimes referred to as the 'Children's Charter', carried out a major revision of existing legislation relating to children and introduced a variety of measures for their legal protection. Parents who ill-treated or neglected their children could now be prosecuted. Foster parents now had to be officially registered with their local authority. The Act also banned the sale of cigarettes to children, their visiting pubs and pawnbrokers, and their employment in dangerous trades like the scrap metal industry.

Children who broke the law were now dealt with by special juvenile courts. However, the 1908 Act still maintained the distinction between Reformatory and Industrial Schools. Reformatory Schools continued to receive youthful offenders below the age of 16, while Industrial Schools received children under 14 found to be destitute, begging or wandering the streets, or whose parents were deemed unfit to look after them, or who associated with reputed thieves or prostitutes. The Act included a provision for children to be transferred between the two types of school. A period of probation, supervised by a probation officer, became available as an alternative to being sent to an Industrial School.

The *Akbar* Scandal

What proved to be one of the biggest blows to the reputation of the Reformatory School system came in October 1910, when the weekly magazine *John Bull* published an article headlined 'Reformatory School Horrors – How Boys at the Akbar School are Tortured – Several Deaths'. The allegations came from Ronald Adams, the former deputy superintendent at the *Akbar* Nautical Training School at Heswall, near Liverpool. Adams claimed that boys were gagged with blankets before being birched with hawthorn branches, that boys who were ill were caned as malingerers, and that punishments for trivial misdemeanours included being drenched with cold water or being made to stand up all night. It was further alleged that several boys had died as a result of such punishments. A subsequent Home Office investigation by Under-Secretary C. F. G. Masterman rejected all the charges although found that there had been instances of 'irregular punishments'. The inquiry accepted the explanation of the School's principal, Captain Beuttler, that the gagging of boys being caned was purely to prevent their cries disturbing passers-by on the nearby towpath. *John Bull* stood its ground, calling Masterman's report a 'white-washing' and claiming that staff at the school who had spoken out against Captain Beuttler had been threatened by a Home Office inspector. Eventually, Home Secretary Winston Churchill appointed a departmental committee to conduct a broad review of Reformatories and Industrial Schools.

Further press condemnation of Reformatories appeared the following year in a series of six articles in the *Daily Mail* which claimed that they were 'Schools for Crime'. Among the *Mail's* allegations were that the boys lacked proper supervision, and were supervised by men who had no training in prison routine. The fact that the Reformatories and Industrial Schools were predominantly run by voluntary rather than state organizations was also criticized. In 1911, none of the existing thirty-seven Reformatories in England and Wales was run by a local authority, and only twenty-two of the 112 Industrial Schools.[19]

In the wake of all the bad publicity, committals to Reformatory and Industrial Schools declined steeply and a number of institutions were forced to close. Eventually, in 1925, the Home Office set up a departmental committee to examine the future of the Schools. Its report, issued in 1927, recommended that the distinction between Reformatory and Industrial Schools be abolished and replaced by a single type of establishment, to be known as the Approved School, which would cater for 'all classes of neglected and delinquent children'.[20] The term 'delinquent' was specified as any young person under the age of 17 who was proved to have committed any offence. The basis for a child being 'neglected' broadly continued on the principles embodied in the 1908 Children Act and included children found begging, wandering or destitute, children whose parents were unfit to care for them because of criminal or drunken habits, children associating or living with prostitutes, and so on. The report also suggested the addition of children 'falling into bad associations, or [who] are exposed to moral danger or are beyond control', and those against whom specified offences, such as cruelty or sexual offences, were committed, or who were living in homes where such offences had been committed against other children.

The Committee's recommendations came into effect through the 1932 Children and Young Persons Act (slightly revised as part of the 1933 Children and Young Persons Act). Following the Act, most of the existing Reformatory and Industrial schools converted to what then became known as Approved Schools.

Chapter 3

Approved Schools

The 1933 Children and Young Persons Act provided a number of alternative courses of action for what were now described as 'juveniles in need of care or protection' and 'juvenile offenders', including being sent to an Approved School, put on probation, or put into the care of 'any fit person' – a role which could also be assumed by a local authority. Courts could, in addition, sentence male juvenile offenders to be 'privately whipped with not more than six strokes of a birch rod by a constable'. A child could be admitted to an Approved School if he or she:

- Was found guilty of an offence which, in the case of an adult, would be punishable by a prison sentence.
- Was found to be in need of care, protection or control.
- Was deemed to be 'refractory' while in the care of a Local Authority.
- Was brought back to Court because of behaviour while on probation.
- Had run away from the care of a Local Authority or a 'fit person'.
- Had come before the Court for truancy.

Children up to the age of 16 could be committed to an Approved School, rather than the previous upper limit that had existed of fifteen. The maximum length of sentence was now three years.

As under the previous system, inmates of Approved Schools could be released on licence. However, details such as the minimum period to be spent at a School before this was allowed, or whether the licence should have a fixed duration, were not specified in the Act.

The 1933 Act also introduced a requirement for local authorities to provide Remand Homes. The Homes, first introduced by the 1901 Youthful Offenders Act, were intended to provide safe custody for young people, between the ages of 8 and 16 inclusive, temporarily being held in custody, for example awaiting a court hearing or transfer to an Approved School.

Types of Approved School

Approved Schools were divided into categories based on the age range of the children they dealt with. The Approved Schools for boys were divided into Senior (aged 15 to 16), Intermediate (13 to 14) and Junior (under 13). Initially, the Approved Schools for Girls were specified as Senior (15 to 16) and Junior (under 15), although an Intermediate category was subsequently introduced. The Junior boys' category was also later split into Primary (up to 10½) and Secondary (10½ to 13). Most of the existing Reformatory and Industrial Schools converted to become Approved Schools and so the great majority of the institutions continued to be operated by voluntary bodies. When the new system was introduced in 1933–4, there were initially eighty-six establishments in England and Wales, mostly former Industrial Schools. By 1938, there were 104 Approved Schools housing a total of 7,268 boys and 1,496 girls. Most of the additional establishments were for girls.[1] Between 1933 and 1950, a total of fifty new Approved Schools were established.[2]

A significant factor in the increase in demand for Approved School places was the raising of the age limit for committals to 16, with a

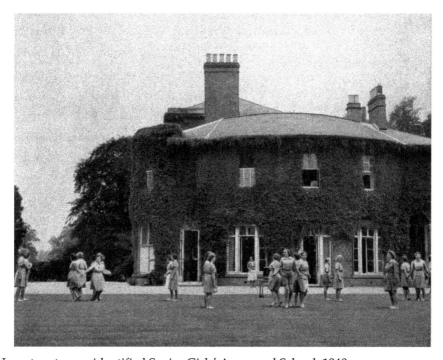

Inmates at an unidentified Senior Girls' Approved School, 1940s.

similar change being made in the upper age of cases dealt with by the juvenile courts. This resulted in an increase in the proportion of Approved School inmates who were offenders. Under the previous system, in 1924, it had been 24 per cent. By 1936, the figure had risen to 78 per cent. From the late 1930s through to around 1950, there was a surge in juvenile delinquency which fuelled an increase in the Approved School population. The particular increase in the number of girls committed was explained by a 1951 Home Office report:

> As the possibilities of action under the care or protection provisions of the Children and Young Persons Act came to be realized by local authorities and the courts, immoral girls aged 16 were brought before the juvenile courts in increasing numbers. Furthermore, war-time influences, including the presence of foreign troops in this country, led to a still greater increase in the number of girls of 15 and 16 falling into immoral ways.[3]

As if to underline the point, a number of the girls' establishments now provided facilities for the treatment of venereal disease.

A further development of came in 1943 when Aycliffe Approved School became the first Classifying School. Previously, magistrates had named a specific Approved School when committing a child to confinement. The role of the Classifying School was to assess the 'character, mental attainments and physical abilities' of new entrants into the Approved School system and decide which institution would then best meet their needs. After the Second World War, four more Classifying Schools were established for boys and two for girls.

Scandals and Crises

As had previously happened with Reformatories, the standing of the Approved School was eroded over the years by a number of scandals and crises which eventually proved fatal for the system.

At the start of 1947, serious discontent began to brew among the boys at the Standon School in Staffordshire, run by the Church of England Children's Society (formerly the Waifs and Strays Society). Some of this was due to the school's isolated rural location and the inadequacy of its sports and recreation facilities, all of which had been exacerbated by a long spell of bad weather. There was also increasing ill-feeling towards the headmaster, Thomas Dawson, particularly over his reluctance to review the readiness of older boys to be released on licence, apparently because their loss from the school roll would cause difficulties in the viability of certain of the school's activities. Dawson had also earned resentment for his restrictions on how the boys used their weekly pocket money, and his imposition of collective fines and punishments for misdemeanours had caused bitterness among those who were innocent.

The unrest came to a head on Saturday, 15 February 1947, when shocking events took place that led to the school's closure. A group of nine boys, who had developed a considerable grudge against the headmaster, decided to kill him and then to abscond in his car after robbing the school's safe and stores. They broke into the school's cadet force armoury and took three rifles, having stolen some poorly secured ammunition from Dawson's quarters the previous day. During their preparations for the attack, however, the boys were discovered by an assistant master, Peter Fieldhouse. One of the group, Gerald Cawley, aged 15, fired several shots at Fieldhouse, inflicting grievous wounds from which he died half an hour later. Panicked by the shooting, the boys made their escape from the school through deep snow, taking the rifles with them, but they were all recaptured a few hours later. Four of

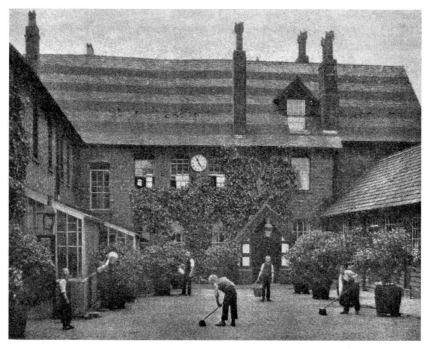

The Standon Farm School, forced to close after the murder of a teacher by an inmate in 1947.

the boys were subsequently found guilty of Fieldhouse's murder and ordered to be detained during His Majesty's pleasure. Five other boys pleaded guilty of a charge of conspiracy to murder.

A subsequent parliamentary Committee of Inquiry into the events at Standon made a number of general recommendations about the management and inspection of Approved Schools, the licensing of pupils, the storage and use of weapons and ammunition, and the provision of recreational activities. With regard to Standon Farm School in particular, the Committee recommended that the headmaster be dismissed and that the school should be closed. As a result of the bad publicity surrounding the events at the Standon School, the reputation of the Waifs and Strays Society was badly dented.

In August 1959, a serious disturbance occurred at the Carlton Approved School, near Bedford, when several groups of boys openly rebelled against the institution's staff. They instigated a mass absconding and invited the press to come and report on their grievances against the staff and headmaster. Their complaints included ill-treatment by staff, unduly long detention at the school before they were released on licence, the withholding of their mail and delays in dispatching outgoing mail.

A subsequent inquiry by Victor Durand QC found that some of these accusations were justified. Its report concluded that some staff had regularly administered illicit punishments. It also found that the headmaster had been detaining the boys longer than normal, claiming that was in an attempt to improve the success rate of the school. The complaints about mail had some foundation but were largely due to mismanagement rather than deliberate policy. The Durand Report resulted and recommended a number of changes in the Approved School system, including the provision of secure units or secure rooms for very difficult boys, the provision of more accommodation within the system, and improvement in officers' salaries in order to attract better quality staff.

The scandal that really spelled the end for the Approved School system broke in March 1967 at the Court Lees School in Surrey. It followed the publication in the *Guardian* of an anonymous letter from a teacher at an unnamed boys' Approved School, expressing his concerns about the state of affairs at the establishment. He claimed that he frequently heard boys screaming while being punished, and that pupils and staff were on the verge of revolt. The *Daily Mail* then printed photographs of the badly bruised bottoms of boys from the school, again supplied by the author of the *Guardian* letter. An investigation by the Home

Office soon determined that the school in question was Court Lees and that the letter writer was named Ivor Cook. An official inquiry ascertained that the school's headmaster had broken Approved School rules on corporal punishment in a number of respects. He had been very free with his use of the cane, sometimes as the initial response to misbehaviour. His cane exceeded the authorized thickness, and boys being caned had been made to remove their trousers. Punishments on a few occasions had been excessively severe, and on many occasions had not been recorded in the school's punishment book. Following the report, the then Home Secretary, Roy Jenkins, ordered the dismissal of the Headmaster and his Deputy, and the closure of the school.

The lengthy controversy stirred up by the events at Court Lees undoubtedly played its part in the decision in 1969 to replace Approved Schools by a new type of institution, the Community Home with Education (CHE), for which local councils had the major responsibility.

Community Homes with Education

The 1969 Children and Young Persons Act introduced major changes in the way that children who were neglected or in trouble were dealt with. The intention of the Act was 'to create a fundamental change in the care and treatment of children and young persons by breaking down the discrimination in attitude and care towards offenders, and others with behavioural difficulties or social disadvantage'. Juvenile delinquency came to be seen as a symptom of deprivation which required treatment rather than punishment.[4]

The Act aimed to create a system of care whereby local authorities provided a range of services oriented to keeping children away from custodial establishments and maintaining them in the community. The legislation gave a much greater role to local authorities in this matter and correspondingly reduced the involvement of central government. Previously, courts had been able to make an Approved School Order to specify that an individual should be committed to such an establishment. Now, children were placed in the hands of the local authority to decide the most appropriate way that they should be dealt with.

The most visible effect of the Act was the abolition of the system of Approved Schools that had been operating since 1933, and the creation of new Community Homes with Education (CHEs). As their name implies, the new homes provided education on the premises for those who could not make use of normal community facilities. Although local authorities could establish their own CHEs, virtually all of them were conversions of former Approved Schools, most of which were run by voluntary bodies – either national organizations such as Barnardo's or the committees of local charities. Under the new arrangements, a voluntary CHE could be either 'Assisted', largely retaining its independence and charging a local authority for the service it provided, or 'Controlled', with the authority running the home, while the voluntary body retained ownership of the property and had some share in its management.

The remit of the CHEs was not specifically to house children identified as 'delinquents' but to provide for those 'who present anti-social and aggressive behaviour and whose disturbance is such that it calls for particular investigation and treatment'.[5]

As well as the CHEs, hundreds of other 'ordinary' Community Homes were established by the conversion of former remand homes, children's homes and nurseries. The particular title of Community Home with Education was, semi-officially at least, used to distinguish former Approved Schools from the other new Community Homes.

By 1977, 110 CHEs were in operation, housing around 7,000 children. By 1990, only twenty-three remained, with 1,149 children in residence.[6] The decline mirrored the general downward trend in all forms of children's residential care and a move towards community-based care such as fostering, supplemented by specialist provision for those with special needs such behavioural or emotional problems. The relatively high cost of running CHEs was also an important factor in the many closures that took place.

In Scotland, a slightly different scheme was introduced by the 1968 Social Work Act, which aimed to bring Approved Schools under the control of local authority social work departments. As a result of a title in a list drawn up by the Scottish Education Department, the former Approved Schools in Scotland became known as 'List D' schools.

Secure Homes

In response to the decline in CHEs, the continuing need for custodial accommodation for the young was met by the 1989 Children Act. The legislation provided for local authorities to establish secure children's homes for children and young people who had absconded from other forms of accommodation, or whose behaviour was judged by a court to present a significant and immediate threat to their own safety or the safety of others. At the present time there are around fifteen secure homes in operation.

Chapter 4

Training Ships

The earliest naval training ships were run by the Marine Society, founded in 1756 by the energetic Jonas Hanway, who was also a governor of the London Foundling Hospital and promoter of the 1766 Act which removed young children from London workhouses. The Marine Society started life recruiting boys and young men for the Royal Navy at the beginning of the Seven Years' War against France but, in an effort to reduce desertions, began training its boys before they were sent to sea. In 1786, the Society purchased a merchant ship, the *Beatty*, which was converted to a training ship and renamed *Marine Society*. In 1876, the Society acquired the training ship *Warspite*, whose intake included boys placed by the workhouse authorities. By 1911, the Society had sent 65,667 men and boys to sea, of which 28,538 had gone into the Royal Navy.

The Royal Navy's own first training ship, established in 1855, was HMS *Implacable* in Plymouth, followed by HMS *Illustrious* in Portsmouth. The ships aimed to give a training in naval life, skills, and discipline to teenage boys – or 'lads' as they were invariably called – and, of course, provide a ready source of recruits for Her Majesty's ships. Over the next fifty years, around thirty other training ships were set up by a variety of other organizations, both public and private, and catering for boys from a wide range of backgrounds, not just the orphaned and homeless. Some, like the *Warspite* and *Arethusa* were charitably-run institutions aimed at helping the children of the poor. Others ranged from those for fee-paying prospective naval officers on the *Worcester* and *Conway*, through to those in Poor Law or other institutional care such as the *Goliath* and *Exmouth*. A number of ships served as Industrial Schools, e.g. the *Shaftesbury* on the Thames at Grays, and the *Clio* on the Menai Straits, or as Reformatories, e.g. the *Cornwall* on the Thames at Purfleet, and the *Akbar* on Merseyside. The *Clarence*, also on Mersey, was used as a Reformatory for Roman Catholic boys.

Boys typically joined the ships at the age of 11 or 12 and stayed until they were 15 or sixteen. Discipline aboard the ships was strict and the birch often used to enforce it. On the *Shaftesbury*, boys were only issued with boots after they had been on board for at least six

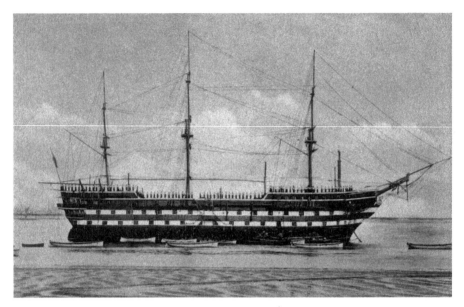

The Training Ship *Exmouth*, established in 1877, was moored on the Thames at Grays, Essex, to provide nautical training to boys placed by the workhouse authorities.

months, by which time they were considered less likely to run away.[1] Food was limited in quantity and variety – biscuit, potatoes and meat were the staples, with occasional green vegetables. Many of the new boys could not swim and needed to be taught – unfortunately some drowned before they mastered the skill. Sleeping accommodation was usually in hammocks, which could be comfortable in the summer but icy-cold in winter.

As well as learning nautical skills such as navigation, sail-making and telegraphy, boys on training ships could learn other useful crafts including tailoring, shoemaking, carpentry and cookery. Training ships usually had a military band where boys with any musical inclinations could develop their talents.

Several boys' establishments, located away from the sea, set up fully rigged masts on which nautical training could be given. In the case of Quarriers' Homes in Bridge of Weir, Renfrewshire, a complete sailing ship, the *James Arthur*, funded by a Clydeside ship-builder, was cemented into the ground in 1887. A full-time sea captain was appointed to teach thirty of the boys seafaring skills.

Training Ships could be dangerous places, however, with several suffering disastrous accidents. In September 1870, a boat belonging

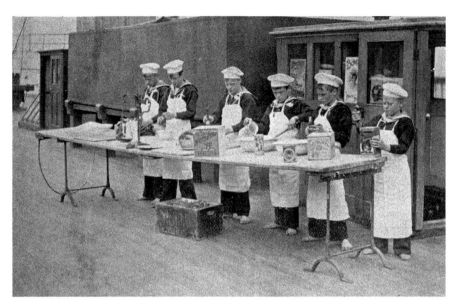

Boys learning to cook aboard the Training Ship *Wellesley*. The vessel, moored on the Tyne at North Shields from 1874, was run by a charity set up by local businessmen.

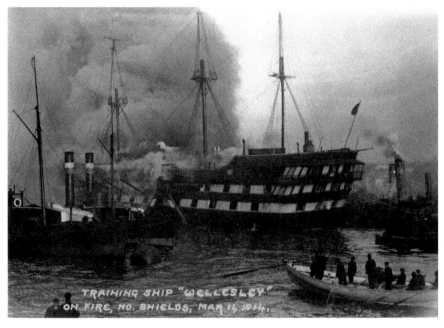

The *Wellesley* was destroyed by a fire on 11 March 1914. It was subsequently re-established as the land-based Wellesley Nautical School in Blyth.

to the *Chichester* was cut in two by a steamer off Greenhithe, resulting in the death of four of the *Chichester* boys. In August 1915, sixteen boys and an officer died after the sailing cutter *Alert*, belonging to the *Cornwall*, collided with a steam tug on the Thames at Purfleet.

Fire was a particular hazard aboard wooden vessels, and a number of the ships met their demise through burning. In December 1875, the *Goliath*, moored on the Thames off Grays, was destroyed by fire, with the loss of twenty-three lives. The fire began in the ship's lamp room, when a cadet accidentally dropped a lamp. Arson by a ship's inmates also resulted in several sinkings. Particularly notorious was the *Clarence*, which regularly suffered from indiscipline and even mutiny on several occasions. On 17 January 1884, at around 1.30 p.m., a fire was discovered in the bows of the ship in an area where oil cans were stored. The vessel sank the next day, with all the inmates having been safely evacuated. Seven of the boys were later found guilty of having set fire to the ship and received five years' penal servitude. Somewhat reluctantly, the Admiralty provided a replacement vessel. However, fire struck again in the early hours of 26 July 1899, when the ship's occupants included the Bishop of Shrewsbury who was on board to perform a confirmation ceremony later that day. As before, the fire had been started on purpose. For several weeks, some of the boys had been stockpiling old rags and other flammable material in the depths of the hold. The fire had been lit deliberately to coincide with the Bishop's visit to the ship.

With the advent of steam power, naval crews became smaller and the demand for boys steadily declined, particularly in the Merchant Service. Many of the original wooden training ships also became unseaworthy and their operation gradually moved onto land-based premises. Some survived until the end of the twentieth century but were then forced to close by a reduction in demand for places and in their funding.

Chapter 5

The Shaftesbury Homes and 'Arethusa'

The Ragged School movement spawned an important organization which, for much of its history, was known as the Shaftesbury Homes and 'Arethusa'. Now known as Shaftesbury Young People, the charity operated under a variety of names over the years, some rather cumbersome, and for simplicity will here be generally referred to as the Society.

Origins

The Society had its origins in the work of a solicitor's clerk named William Williams. In 1843, on a train journey from Paddington to the West Country, Williams's attention was caught by a noisy group of boys who, he discovered, were cold, dirty, miserable, chained together, and being transported to Australia as convicts. Determined to do something to help the plight of such boys, he founded a ragged school in the St Giles-in-the-Fields district of London – one the dirtiest, roughest and most crowded parts of the capital.

The school was successful and in 1844 joined with a number of others to form an umbrella organization, the Ragged School Union. Later that year, the Right Honourable Lord Ashley, MP (known as the Earl of Shaftesbury from 1851), became the Union's president. He soon met William Williams and the two became good friends.

The Streatham Street School's Committee was constantly on the lookout for larger and more suitable premises, although this proved difficult, partly because of landlords' reluctance to take on such tenants, but also because large sections of St Giles were being demolished and redeveloped. In 1848, the School was forced temporarily to share premises with the Irish Free School in George Street, St Giles. In 1850, it merged with two other ragged schools in a similar situation, one located at Abbey Place, Little Coram Street, the other in the very disreputable location of Neal's Yard. The new grouping was known as The St Giles and St George, Bloomsbury, Ragged Schools. In an effort to rationalize its operation, the Society raised money to buy permanent

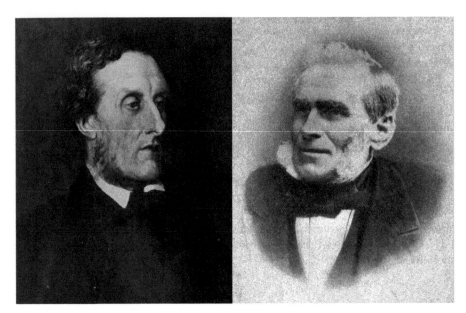

Lord Shaftesbury (left) and William Williams, the two leading figures in the Ragged School movement.

premises and acquired a property at 19 Broad Street, Bloomsbury. Formerly used as a 'gin palace', the building comprised four storeys plus a basement, with plenty of space for separate schoolrooms for boys, girls and infants, plus residential refuge accommodation for up to a hundred children.

In 1853, the Neal's Yard premises were converted for use as a night refuge for homeless boys who were fed and given a bed but had to fend for themselves in the daytime. Those who demonstrated a willingness to learn were transferred to Broad Street when places became available. Reflecting the broadening of its scope, the Society now became the St Giles and St George, Bloomsbury, Refuge for Destitute Children and Ragged and Industrial Schools.

From 1855, only girls were housed at Broad Street, with a separate refuge for boys being opened at Arthur Street, St Giles. A new home for the older girls from Broad Street was opened in Acton in 1860, and provided a laundry service for all the Society's other establishments. The Acton home relocated to Ealing in 1867.

In 1857, the boys' refuge at Arthur Street moved to larger premises – a former coach factory on Great Queen Street. The sum of £850 needed to alter and equip the building included a grant from the Ragged School Union, and funds raised by Lord Ashley.

Emigration

Almost from the outset, the Society used emigration as a way of ensuring the future employment prospects for its children. In June 1848, Lord Ashley made a speech in the House of Commons suggesting that an annual government grant be made to fund the voluntary emigration of children from London's ragged schools. His proposal received widespread support and the sum of £1,500 was subsequently made available for the purpose.

At the end of 1848, a party of twenty-two boys became the first to emigrate under the scheme, each of them having been provided by the Society with a new outfit of clothes and a Bible. In all, 134 boys and sixteen girls, selected from among 6,000 at thirty different ragged schools, departed to begin new lives in New South Wales. Although the government grant was not renewed, the Society carried on funding the passage each year of as many children as it could afford.

In 1883, a house in Hamilton, Ontario, was taken by the Society on a three-year lease as a reception home for its boys who were emigrating to Canada. It provided a base for new arrivals until they found a job, and also a temporary home for those who were out of work or ill. Financial and other difficulties led to its move to cheaper premises in nearby Wingham and eventual closure in 1888.

Also in 1888, Lord Jersey came to see off that season's party of the Society's boys travelling to Canada and donated a sovereign to each, payable once they had commenced their new employment. The following year, a party of twenty-four boys emigrated under the care of a Mr William J. Pady who assured the Society that they had all been found suitable employment. Pady organized emigration parties for a number of organizations but was later revealed as a totally disreputable character. His supposed receiving home in Canada was actually his brother's small farm shack, and the children he escorted were often under-equipped for the harsh winters they were to face. The Children's Aid Society subsequently described Pady as a 'slimy scoundrel'.[1]

The *Chichester* and *Arethusa*

In 1866, Lord Shaftesbury, as he had now become known, became the Society's Patron and in the same year launched a new initiative to take boys off the streets by giving them a training for a life at sea. On 14 February, St Valentine's Night, he organized a supper at the Broad Street Refuge to which were invited any boys under the age of 16 who were staying at night refuges and workhouse casual wards (vagrants' overnight accommodation) in the area. Tempted by the prospect of a warm fire and free hot meal, around 200 boys overcame their natural caution and attended the event. After the visitors had been filled up with roast beef, plum pudding and coffee, Lord Shaftesbury spent some time going around the room, talking the boys and hearing about their lives.

He then addressed the assembled company. 'Supposing that there were in the Thames a big ship, large enough to contain a thousand boys, would you like to be placed on board to be taught trades or trained for the navy and merchant service?'[2] Shaftesbury's words were greeted with cheers and roars of approval and he promised to set about finding a vessel for the scheme. His request to the Admiralty received a rapid and positive response, with the redundant frigate *Chichester* being offered for the purpose. After being fitted out, the *Chichester* was moored on the Thames off Greenhithe and officially inaugurated into its new role on 18 December 1866.

The *Chichester* proved a great success with more than 1,300 boys accepted for training on the ship by the summer of 1874, up to 250 being resident on board at any one time. A proposal to establish a second ship was quickly met by the offer of £5,000 from Lady Burdett-Coutts to fund the venture. The Admiralty again proved forthcoming and provided the *Arethusa*, a wooden frigate accommodating 250 boys, which was also moored at Greenhithe.

Life Aboard the *Chichester* and *Arethusa*

The *Chichester's* first Commanding Officer was the recently retired Captain A. H. Alston who, although a devout Christian, was a stern disciplinarian. Other staff included William McCarthy as Chief Officer, Mr Phillips as Schoolmaster, and Messrs William Samuels and J. Marsh as Instructors – all lived on board and worked a seven-day week. Mrs McCarthy, the Chief Officer's wife, was awarded £20 per year for teaching the boys how to cut out and make their own clothes from material supplied by the Naval Yard at Deptford. However, both she and her husband were dismissed for drunkenness in January 1868.

An early task was teaching the boys to swim, although sadly there were several instances of boys falling overboard and drowning. To help with this problem, a barge was moored to the head of the ship and filled with water to act as makeshift swimming pool. By the end of

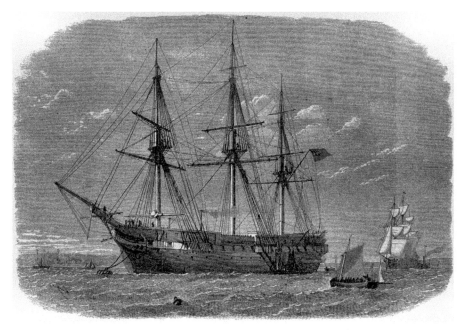

The Training Ship *Chichester* was moored on the Thames at Greenhithe from 1867.

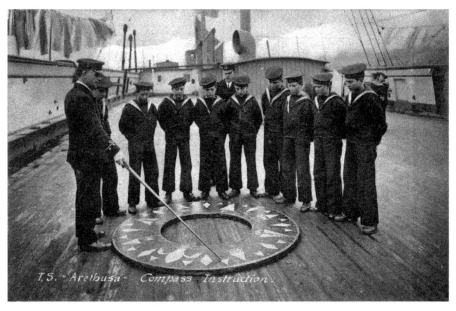

Compass instruction aboard the Training Ship *Arethusa*.

the first year 184 boys had been received on the ship. Of the forty-two who had moved on, twenty-one were placed in merchant ships, nine entered the Royal Navy, seven returned ashore, one became apprenticed to a tailor, two had drowned and one had died of fever.[3]

Training on the *Chichester* included the use of compass and lead, knotting and splicing, sail-making, knowledge of all running gear and parts of the ship, reefing and furling sails, and rowing and steering, not to mention time spent in swimming, cooking, carpentry and tailoring.

In April 1869, increasing friction between Captain Alston and the ship's governing committee over matters such as his being allowed to have a wine cellar on board, led to his being called upon to resign. However, Alston took his revenge by persuading all the ship's instructors to depart with him to positions on another vessel.

Misdemeanours by the inmates resulted in a birching, which could only be administered by the Captain. The birching scale ranged from twenty-four cuts and dismissal with disgrace for any act of gross indecency or immoral behaviour, to twelve cuts and dismissal for stealing, and six cuts for being in an improper place. Absconding earned twelve cuts, although a second offence brought dismissal from the ship.[4]

Originally, the boys were known on board only by their number – when they met up in later life, none of them knew each other's names. This custom was to continue until 1927, after which time boys were referred to by their surnames.

The boys' food was limited in both quantity and variety. The daily dietary scale for many years comprised:

1lb soft bread
8oz biscuit
7oz fresh meat
8oz potatoes
¾oz cocoa
⅛oz tea
⅔oz sugar

There were also occasional green vegetables and twice-weekly rations of pea soup and rice, with treacle pudding as a treat on Sundays.

Moving Out of London

Once the *Chichester* had come into service, the Society began to look for accommodation in the countryside, to which boys could be moved from the slums of London. In 1867, a farm for sale was found in Bisley, near Woking in Surrey, and fund-raising began to purchase the property and erect the required premises. The establishment, which became the Society's Farm School and Country Home, began operation in 1868. Bisley could accommodate 150 boys who were taught farming skills, carpentry, tailoring and bread-making. Some also learned telegraphy, a skill then becoming much in demand in the commercial world. And like many boys' institutions, the School also had its own uniformed wind band. In 1873, the accommodation at Bisley was increased by the construction of a second home in the grounds of the Farm School, which was named the Shaftesbury School.

In 1872, the girls from the Broad Street refuge moved to a more rural location at Sudbury Hall, Wembley. The Broad Street premises were then converted to a lodging house for working boys. In 1878, the boys' refuge in Great Queen Street relocated to a large mansion in Twickenham, known as Fortescue House.

The End of the Ragged Schools

The 1870 Elementary Education Act introduced a system of School Boards to supplement the existing voluntary provision for children aged for 5 to 13 years. A Board could be set up in any area where the existing number of school places was calculated to be insufficient. Board Schools were funded by local rates and could also charge weekly attendance fees, although children from poor families could be admitted without payment. From 1880, school attendance was made compulsory for all those aged 5 to 13, and in 1891 all public elementary schools became free.

A significant effect of the 1870 and later Acts was steadily to reduce the need for ragged schools. This was implicitly acknowledged by the Society in 1872 when its name was changed to the National Refuges for Homeless and Destitute Children and 'Chichester' Training Ship. The last ragged school, being run by the Society in Little Coram Street, was finally closed in 1891 after forty-five years of operation. A few ragged schools continued in operation into the twentieth century, with the last thought to have closed in around 1910.

In 1871, the Society began an experiment in the shape of the Newsboys' Home at 80 Gray's Inn Road. The Home, which was superintended by a married couple, offered modestly priced bed and board to boys selling newspapers and other articles on the city's streets. In 1875, the establishment began to also offer accommodation to boys starting work in London and so was renamed the Home for Working Boys.

A New Headquarters

In 1886, the Society decided to bring together all its London activities (with the exception of the Little Coram Street Ragged School) at a single location. After no suitable premises could be found, a site was purchased on the recently constructed thoroughfare of Shaftesbury Avenue and an architect was commissioned to design a new building.

On 17 June 1887, the Prince of Wales laid the foundation stone of what was originally to be known as 'The Jubilee Memorial Home' in honour of Queen Victoria's Golden Jubilee. The ceremony was attended by 400 children from the Society's various establishments and music was provided by the boys' band from one of the homes. By the time that the Countess of Jersey formally opened the completed building on 15 May 1888, it had adopted the name Shaftesbury House, with the address of 164 Shaftesbury Avenue. The premises included accommodation for a hundred destitute boys and thirty-five working boys, together with a club, institute and offices for the Society. The working boys' department was renamed Fordham House in 1892 in memory of John Fordham, a long-serving Treasurer of the Society.

In 1896, the boys' refuge at Shaftesbury House was turned into a Technical School for older boys from the Society's other homes. Boys arrived at the age of 14 and received up to two years of instruction in shoemaking or tailoring.

A New Century

Several new fund-raising ventures were launched in 1900. Children from comfortable homes were targeted by the formation of a 'Victoria League' for girls, and an 'Arethusa League' for boys. Lantern-slide presentations of the Society's work were prepared, after which collections were taken. A network of local agents was set up to promote the Society and to receive donations. The Society also benefited from substantial donations from Alfred Fennings, the founder of a successful company selling over-the-counter medicines such as Fennings' Fever Cure. After Fennings's death in 1900, the Society continued to receive the profits from his company which eventually ran into millions of pounds.

On the occasion of its Diamond Jubilee in 1903, the Society decided to set up a new home for girls who were too young to attend the existing establishments at Sudbury and Ealing. Financial constraints delayed progress with the scheme but in 1906 a site was purchased in Royston in Hertfordshire. The Little Girls' Home,

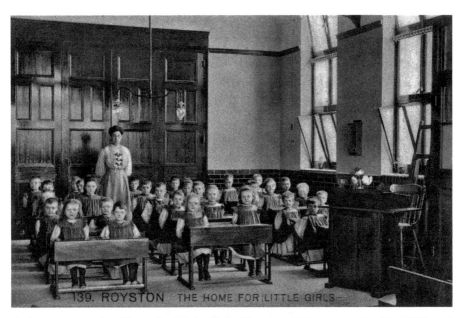

A classroom at the Home for Little Girls, Royston. It became mixed in 1921 and was boys-only by 1929.

which accommodated up to eighty children, was officially opened in November 1908.

The First World War

The First World War caused great difficulties for the Society. Its income suffered considerably from a substantial fall in donations and by 1916 had a deficit of over £6,000. The *Chichester* was sold off in 1917 for 500 guineas. This, together with a highly successful appeal for funds to city insurance, shipping and marine companies, brought the deficit down to £1,500.

The homes also received gifts of food from as far away as Australia via the London Chamber of Commerce. The donations received by the *Arethusa* included eight cases of preserved meat, four cases of boiled mutton, ten cases of rabbits, four sheep carcasses, twelve bags of sugar, ten sacks of flour, six boxes of butter, twelve cases of syrup and eight cases of jam.[5]

Many of the Society's staff were called up for military duty, result-ing in even more stress for those trying to keep the homes running. Mrs Swaffield, the matron at Sudbury Hall, whose son was a serving officer, could not cope with the strain and suffered repeated health problems because of 'intemperance' and was asked to resign.[6]

A Changing Image

In 1919, the Society's existing name (the National Refuges for Homeless and Destitute Children) was felt to be out of keeping with the times and, it was said, upsetting to many of those in the Society's homes. The new name that was adopted was the Shaftesbury Homes and Arethusa. (In 1944, the Ragged School Union was renamed the Shaftesbury Society but, despite the similarity in names, was always a separate organization from the Shaftesbury Homes.)

Reflecting the change of name, efforts began to make the Society's establishments homelier and less institutional. At the Ealing girls' home, greater contact with the local community was encouraged and a Girl Guides company started.

The employment prospects of the children also received increasing attention. For the boys, in particular, an increasingly wide range of occupations was becoming available. For girls, however, although nursing and teaching offered an alternative to domestic employment, there were some in the Society who were concerned at the 'over-education of the working classes'. At a conference of the Society's Ladies' Association in 1926, one speaker saw the ideal destination for many girls as the 'good wives' of the 'splendid young men of the Dominions'.[7]

New Homes for Old

In 1929, the Society took over the Newport Market Army Training School, founded in 1863 at Newport Market, Soho, to train poor boys for a career as military bandsmen. Under the Society's control, the School – then based at Orpington – was renamed The Newport Market Army Bands School.

Also in 1929, increasing structural problems with the building at the Sudbury Hall girls' home led to a search for new premises. The following year, the Society acquired Esher Place in Surrey, a large mansion set in ten acres of grounds. The property was large enough to also accommodate the girls from the Ealing home. Most of the £8,000 cost of converting Esher Place was raised by the sale of the Sudbury Hall and Ealing House properties. At around this time, the Royston establishment was turned into a home for young boys.

The venerable *Arethusa* came to the end of her life in 1932 when she was condemned as unfit for further service. She was replaced by the *Peking*, a steel-hulled barque built in Hamburg in 1911. Renamed *Arethusa*, the vessel was refitted at the Royal Dockyard, Chatham, and

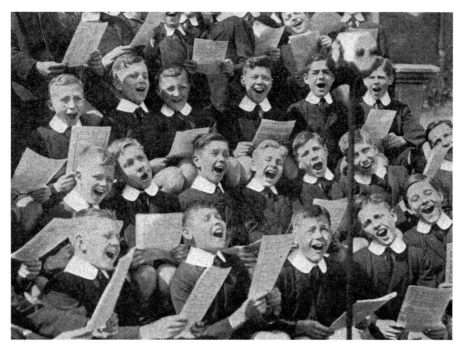

Boys from Fortescue House, Twickenham, in full voice, 1930s.

in July 1933 took up a new mooring on the River Medway at Upnor, near Rochester.

In 1935, following an approach from the National Society for the Protection of Young Girls (Princess Louise Home), which was in financial difficulties, a merger was agreed between the two organizations. The girls' home was then renamed Esher Place (Princess Louise Home for Girls).

In 1937, the Fortescue House boys' home in Twickenham moved to larger premises in the same town – the former Metropolitan and City Police Orphanage, where the Newport Market Army Bands School could also be accommodated. The new establishment had the rather cumbersome official name of Fortescue House (incorporating the Newport Market Army Bands School).

The Second World War

As had happened in 1914–18, the Second World War put a great strain on the Society's operations. Donations and subscriptions were significantly reduced, the prices of food and clothing increased, and extra expenditure was required for matters such as the provision of air-raid shelters and the evacuation of some of the children. Wherever possible, children were returned to their own parents to make room for those who were made homeless or orphaned by the war. Between 1939 and 1941, the number of children in the Society's care fell from 1,200 to 800.

At the Fordham House Hostel in London, the building was reinforced and sleeping accommodation for boys and staff set up in a locker room and adjoining lobby, with the women sleeping in the swimming bath. Underground shelters were set up at the Bisley, Esher and Fortescue House homes.

The Society's homes all contributed to the war effort by growing vegetables on any land they had available. At Royston and Esher, the children picked herbs for food and wild plants for medicine. At Fortescue House and Bisley, the boys made small lathe-turned parts for use by the forces.

After an incendiary bomb landed in the grounds of Esher House, the girls and their teachers were evacuated to a school in Bradford. Two flying bombs fell on Fortescue House in 1944, one on a playing field, the other directly on the building. The boys were subsequently evacuated, some to South Wales, the others to a Nissen-hut camp in Bucklesham in Suffolk. All the boys were later transferred to Pontefract in Yorkshire. The only home to be entirely undamaged was Royston, but not a single child or member of staff was injured in any of the homes.

The Post-War Years

The war had created considerable upheavals for children, especially those without families, and there was growing concern about their situation – no doubt heightened by the major welfare reforms that were in progress at the time. Following the death of a 13-year-old boy, Dennis O'Neill, who in January 1945 was beaten and starved to death by his foster father, the Curtis Committee was appointed to consider how best to make provision for children deprived of a normal home life or parental care. The Committee's report recommended adoption or fostering as the best options, with institutional care, if needed, being in small homes of no more than twelve children. Children in such establishments should be encouraged to maintain contact with relatives and to develop friendships outside the home. The Curtis Report's proposals formed the basis of the 1948 Children Act.

An early sign of the changing approach came in the summer of 1946. The parents of those children in the Society's care who could afford to pay for their fare went home for the holiday. Others spent time in the homes of volunteer 'aunts and uncles'.

The Society also had to contend with the requirements of the 1944 Education Act, under which primary and secondary education was to be provided at separate schools. This caused problems at Bisley where the two original schools had merged in 1919, one becoming the junior department, the other the senior. It was eventually determined that Bisley would have to become a secondary school for boys aged 11 and over, while Fortescue House in Twickenham would be a primary school for those aged 7 to eleven.

In November 1945, the boys at Fordham House moved to larger premises in Hampstead, although the Technical School was discontinued as part of the reorganization. However, the steeply rising costs of the Society's operations – partly due to a post-war surge in the numbers of children being taken into care – meant that cuts had to be made. It was therefore decided in 1948 to close Fordham House. The Society also sold the freehold of its Head Office site on Shaftesbury Avenue, though continued to rent offices on the first floor of the building.

Further retrenchment followed in 1952 with the closure of the Esher Place and Royston homes. Esher Place was replaced by a much smaller house a few miles away in East Molesey. In 1958, Bisley was also closed and the boys transferred to Fortescue House which was reorganized and expanded to create separate junior and senior schools on the same site. On the more positive side, an ocean-going steam yacht, *Glen Strathallan*, was bequeathed to the Society in 1955 for use in the training of boys for the maritime services. It was moored on the Thames alongside the *Arethusa*.

Facing the Future

The Society's financial problems continued into the 1960s. In 1967, its Head Office moved from 164 Shaftesbury Avenue to smaller premises at 229A Shaftesbury Avenue. Its difficulties were added to by the steady trend away from providing residential care in large institutions, which had been the Society's traditional main activity. By the 1970s, there was also a decline in the number of boys interested in training for a life at sea.

In 1972, following a major review by consultants of the Society's options for the future, known as the Hunt Report, three major changes were proposed. First, the *Arethusa* would now be run as a floating secondary boarding school, coupling high-quality education with character training and adventure. Second, the Society would open one or more hostels for homeless school leavers, run along family-style lines. Third, a suitably qualified 'Social Service Secretary' would be appointed to co-ordinate all caring aspects of the Society's work. These recommendations offered a path by which the Society could continue to pursue an active role in the support of young people.

In 1973, the first of the Society's Adolescent Hostels was opened in Putney, housing ten boys in their late teens, under the supervision of a small residential staff. The neighbouring house was subsequently acquired for use as a 'progress' hostel and fitted out as self-contained flatlets for those able to live independently. In 1975, Esher House became a supported hostel for vulnerable, young single mothers with their babies. Funding for these new initiatives came from the sale in 1974 of the Society's last big property, Fortescue House in Twickenham. The remaining residents of Fortescue House were transferred to new premises in Hanworth, Middlesex.

Although the *Arethusa* did see a short period of use as a floating school, the cost of its maintenance, together with £100,000 worth of urgently needed repairs, led to the decision to dispose of the vessel. She was sold in 1975 to the South Street Seaport Museum of New York and restored to her 1911 condition and name, the *Peking*. In the same year, a new 71-foot ketch was acquired to become the third *Arethusa*, itself replaced in 1982 by another purpose-built vessel. The *Arethusa's* onshore buildings were developed into the Upnor Venture Centre. Two other new nautical-related projects were the *John Collett Barge*, a floating school for children from the Borough of Southwark who struggled to cope with mainstream education, and the *Sir Alan Herbert*, a sailing barge used as a mobile adventure centre for inner-city children.

Other new ventures in the 1980s and 1990s included the McAndrew House Family Centre in Clapham for parents having difficulty coping with their children, the Ipswich Young Persons' Support Team providing guidance and support to vulnerable young people in the city, and a scheme to manage residential homes for young people on behalf of the Borough of Wandsworth.

In 2006, the charity changed its working name to Shaftesbury Young People. Its present-day mission statement is 'To support young people in care and in need to find their voice, to be healthy, to learn, develop and achieve and to gain an independent and positive place in society'.

Chapter 6

Müller's Orphan Houses

Many of the best-known names who dedicated their lives to institutions and organizations caring for children made their mark during Queen Victoria's reign. It was at the dawn of this era that George Müller began his work that was to culminate in Britain's largest single-site children's home, with more than 2,000 children in residence.

Müller was born in Prussia in 1805 and came to England in 1829 to work for the London Society for Promoting Christianity Among the Jews. In 1832, now married, he moved to Bristol where he became joint pastor at the George Street Bethesda Chapel. He then founded the Scriptural Knowledge Institution for Home and Abroad, whose aims were to aid Christian schools and missionaries, to distribute the Bible and other Christian works, and to run scripturally-based day and Sunday schools.

Müller's work with destitute children began in 1836 when the idea for an 'Orphan House' that had been forming in his mind started to become reality. With the help of donations of money, household goods and clothing from his supporters, he rented a large house at 6 Wilson Street in the St Paul's district of Bristol. The home, which was just for girls, opened its doors on 11 April and by 18 May twenty-six children were in residence, under the care of a matron and governess. Entry to the home was restricted to destitute children, born in wedlock, both of whose parents were deceased.

Encouraged by the success of the venture, Müller opened several further homes on the same street and by 1843, a total of about 120 places for girls, boys and infants were being provided. During this time, the finances of the homes were often perilously low but donations always seemed to appear at the last moment to keep them running. Müller's lifelong philosophy was that prayer would supply all his needs. Instead of asking for contributions towards his support, he always relied on unsolicited offerings.

In 1845, following complaints from nearby residents about the large numbers of children congregating on Wilson Street, Müller began to think about moving to a new location with purpose-built premises that would house up to 300 children. Despite the great expense such

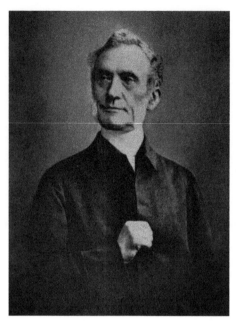

George Müller, founder of the New Orphan Houses, Bristol.

a scheme would involve, a flow of donations soon began to arrive, the first being for £1,000. In February 1846, a seven-acre site was acquired at Ashley Down on the northern side of Bristol, which the owner sold to Müller at a much reduced price for the project. By May 1847, with the total donations having reached £11,000, construction work began. The New Orphan House, as it was originally known, was opened on 18 June 1849 and all the existing children were transferred from Wilson Street. They were joined a few weeks later by 170 new arrivals, with a total of 288 children then in residence. At the same time, a board of eleven trustees was set up to take on legal responsibility for the home and its management.[1]

Not long after the opening of the new home, Müller started to think about increasing the institution's capacity by adding a second and much larger building housing up to 700 children. The proposal was made public in May 1851, with the cost estimated at £27,000 for the land and building, plus about £8,000 for fitting up and furnishing. Money for the new building accumulated slowly at first but was boosted by a number of major individual donations including one of £8,100 in 1853. By mid-1855, the building fund contained over £23,000. A problem arose, however, when it was realized the ground left around the existing house lacked sufficient space for the new building,

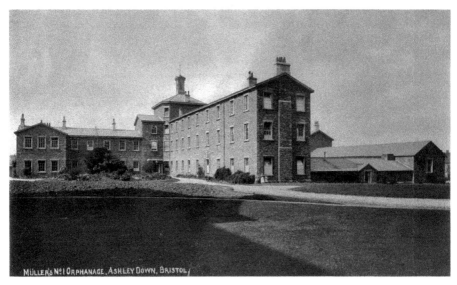

Müller's Orphan House No. 1, opened in 1849.

and the adjoining fields turned out to be unavailable for purchase. Undaunted, Müller revised his plans which were now to include two smaller buildings, one housing 400 children and another for three hundred. Construction work on the first of these began in May 1855 and was completed on 18 September 1857, on which date Müller recorded that he had just tested the new building's 150 gas lamps. The building also had 300 large windows which had been glazed free of charge by a local company. To fit into the available space, the new house had a more linear layout than the original house. The building was occupied by 200 infant girls and 200 older girls.

Construction of the third house, whose 300 places would take the establishment's total capacity to 1,000, became possible in September 1858 when an 11.5-acre site was purchased across the road to the south of the existing buildings. A steady stream of new donations, including one of £7,000 in January 1859, allowed Müller to increase the size of the new block from 300 to 450 places. The building began construction in July 1859 and opened on 12 March 1862. To help the smooth running of the home, older residents from the existing houses were mixed in with the new children.

Even before House No. 3 had opened, Müller was formulating plans for two further blocks whose 850 places would take the site's total capacity to two thousand. The second of these came into use in November 1868.

A Visit to the Homes

A picture of life at the Orphan Homes is provided by the following account of a visit to the establishment in the 1870s:

> *It is a striking sight to watch the Orphans passing through the streets of Bristol, on their way to attend Divine worship. Every Sunday morning they may be seen marching, two and two, up and down the hilly thoroughfares of that ancient city, on their way to Bethesda Chapel, where Mr. Müller ministers. Each Orphan House contributes its troop of two or three hundred children – the boys and girls being marshalled in separate bands, and accompanied by their different masters, matrons, and teachers.*
>
> *The Orphan House No. 1, which contains usually 140 girls above seven years of age, 80 boys of the same age, and 80 infants of either sex, was that that we first visited. There are three school-rooms – Boys', Girls', and Infants' – all large, airy, cheerful-looking apartments. The Girls', which is shown first of the three, is very spacious and lofty, situated on the ground-floor, and well fitted up with the best modern maps and other helps for learning. As our party, numbering some sixty or seventy, entered, we beheld about one hundred and twenty girls, sitting at work at low desks – all clothed alike in blue print frocks and neat pinafores, and with their hair cut short behind, but arranged with the greatest neatness. On a signal from the principal teacher, who was stationed on a small platform, with a desk in front, the girls all stood up and placed their hands behind them. At another signal one of the Orphans struck up a cheerful song, which the rest at once joined in, and all marched out in single file, with as much precision in their steps as any of our modern volunteer corps would exhibit.*
>
> *The Boys' School-room does not materially differ from that of the Girls'. There were, at our entrance, about eighty boys seated at desks, dressed all alike in blue cloth jackets and corduroy trousers. Two separate rooms are appropriated as Work-rooms also – one for the boys, and one for the girls; the former are taught, a few at a time, to knit and mend their own stockings, and the girls to make their own garments, under the superintendence of a teacher who does the cutting out for them. Then come the Play-rooms, one for boys and another for girls. These are large, lofty rooms, with a few low forms, and nothing else in the shape of furniture. These are, of course, only intended for use in bad weather, at least in the case of the boys. For there is a capital court for playing in for each class of Orphans, and swings and other apparatus for exercise and play. The Girls' Play-room was provided with large cupboards, divided into small pigeon-holes, one for each*

child, well stored with dolls, dolls' houses, and a variety of other toys, the gifts, sometimes of relatives (who are allowed to visit the Orphans once a month), sometimes of ladies, who present them to the teachers, to be used as rewards.

The dining room where all the Orphans take their meals is a spacious apartment filled with long narrow tables and forms. While we were inspecting this room, we noticed some of the elder girls employed in spreading the snow-white table-cloths for the evening meal. Others at the same time entered the room with trays loaded with bread-and-butter. Soon afterwards, some hundreds of cups filled with milk-and-water were placed upon the tables; but the Orphans were not called to tea until after the visitors had left.

The food of the Orphans at breakfast is always oatmeal porridge: they use milk with it. No doubt this wholesome food is one cause of the healthy, ruddy appearance of the Orphans generally; for notwithstanding a strong prejudice against it in this country, a more wholesome, nutritious article of diet certainly does not exist. The dinner provided for the children varies almost every day. Monday there is boiled beef; Tuesday, soup, with a good proportion of meat in it; Wednesday, rice-milk with treacle; Thursday they have boiled leg of mutton; the following day they have soup again, and on Saturday bacon; on Sundays they always dine on rice with treacle in order that as few as possible may be kept from attending public worship. The Orphans breakfast at eight o'clock, dine at one, and take tea at six.

Another apartment is called the 'Shoes and Cloak Room'. Every child in the house has three pairs of shoes. The girls all wear cloaks of a green plaid in winter, and shawls in summer. Then there are the 'Washing places'. They are furnished with baths; and all around the walls were hung bags containing the brush and comb belonging to each child, and the number of the said child painted over each.

The children all rise about six o'clock in the morning. They retire to rest – the elder children about eight or nine, the younger an hour earlier. The teachers conduct religious worship every day, at half-past eight in the morning, and just before tea in the afternoon.

As regards the education of the children, the girls are instructed in reading, writing, arithmetic, English grammar, geography, English history, a little of general history, and in all kinds of useful needlework and household work. The boys go through the same course of instruction as the girls, and they learn to knit and mend their own stockings. They also make their beds, clean their shoes, scrub their rooms, and work a little in the garden ground around the Orphan Establishment, in the way of digging, planting, weeding, &c.[2]

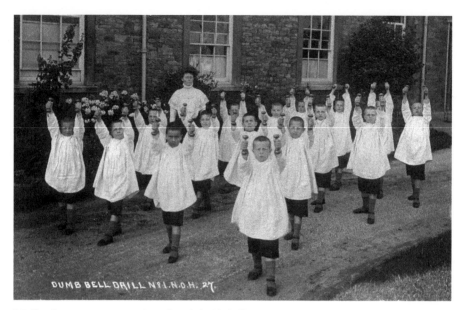

DUMB BELL DRILL N°1. N.O.H. 27.

Müller boys exercise with a dumb-bell drill.

Müller's wife, Mary, died in 1870 and the following year he married Susannah Grace Sanger. In 1875, the couple began a seventeen-year period of missionary travel ranging as far as the USA, India and Australia. With Müller's departure, his son-in-law James Wright took on the position of Director of the homes. In the final years of his life, George Müller lived in No. 3 House and died there on 10 March 1898.

In 1901, following a decline in numbers applying to the orphanage, admission was widened to include 'partial' orphans – those who had lost only one parent.

Gradual improvements to the houses were made over the years, such as the asphalting of the playgrounds and improvements to the water supply, drainage and laundry facilities. In June 1910, a swimming bath was erected between Houses 4 and 5. The bath was closed in 1914, however, after the attendant joined the armed forces, and did not re-open until 1922. The installation of electric lighting in some of the buildings began in 1925.

The occupancy of the houses underwent several changes. At the end of the First World War, part of House No. 1 was converted to a nursery. By the early 1930s, all the boys were living in House No. 4 and a new nursery was opened in No. 3 House.

Unlike many other children's institutions, Müller's made little use of emigration as a way of finding children new homes. In the early

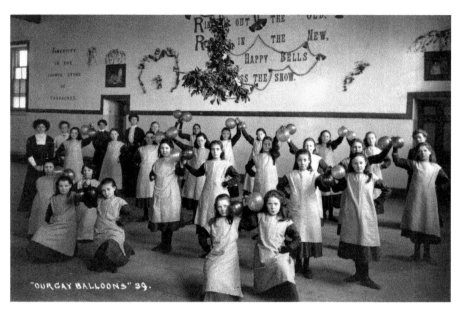

Müller girls pose with festive balloons.

1920s, however, difficulties in finding local employment for the boys led to a small number being sent to work on farms in Canada.

By 1947, the falling number of applicants to the orphanage and the encroachment of the city onto its once semi-rural location had begun to raise doubts about the future of the Ashley Down site. In May of that year, the intake of the homes was widened to include non-orphans. At around the same time, a 400-acre estate was purchased at Backwell Hill, in North Somerset, where – in line with the changing philosophy in children's care – there were plans to establish a new generation of smaller homes. However, the spiralling costs of the scheme led to the estate being sold off in 1957. Instead, it was decided to distribute the remaining children and staff in family-group-style scattered homes in properties purchased in and around Bristol.

In 1958, the charity – then renamed The Müller Homes for Children – finally vacated the Ashley Down site which, during its 109 years of operation, had been home to a total of 11,603 'full' orphans and 5,686 'partial' orphans. The organization moved to much smaller premises at Cotham Park, Bristol, where – now known simply as Müller's – it continues to provide help for those with spiritual and social needs in the UK and beyond.

Chapter 7

Barnardo's Homes

The only other individual who surpassed George Müller in the scale of his achievement was Thomas John Barnardo, a name which was to become virtually synonymous with children's homes. Barnardo was born in Dublin on 4 July 1845, the son of John Barnardo, a Prussian-born furrier, and Abigail O'Brien. The couple had married in 1837 after the death of John's first wife, Elizabeth, who was Abigail's sister and the mother of five young children. The family continued to grow, with Thomas being John and Abigail's fourth son. He proved a somewhat delicate child, and academically bright, though he gained something of a reputation as a troublemaker.

After leaving St Patrick's Cathedral Grammar School, where the brutality of its principal, the Reverend William Dundas, left a considerable impression on Thomas, he worked for four years as an apprentice to a wine merchant. It was during this period, in August 1862, that he underwent a Christian conversion during a religious revival that was sweeping the country. Soon afterwards, he joined the evangelical Plymouth Brethren movement, and then decided to become a candidate for missionary work in China. In 1866, he moved to London to pursue his application for this scheme and to begin studies as a medical student.

Staying in lodgings near Mile End Road in the East End of London, Barnardo witnessed the poverty of many of those living there. He also saw at first hand the effects of a cholera epidemic in the area which killed more than 3,000 people and devastated countless families.

Being judged as unready for the China mission, and unable to register for study at the London Hospital until the autumn of 1867, he made contact with local Plymouth Brethren and began preaching in the streets of Stepney. He also started to teach at the Ernest Street Ragged School and the success of his work soon led to his becoming its superintendent though he fell out with the school's committee and left with the aim of opening his own establishment.

Barnardo was far from being alone in such pursuits. After the 1851 census had indicated that less than half of the population of London's East End could be said to be Christian, the area had become magnet for evangelical groups carrying out mission, 'rescue' and reform work.[1]

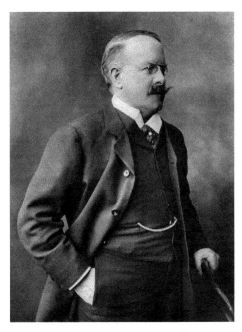

Thomas John Barnardo in about 1900.

The First Home

Barnardo eventually managed to raise the money to rent his first premises at Hope Place, Limehouse, which opened its doors as the East End Juvenile Mission on 2 March 1868. Hope Place was partly a ragged school, providing free classes on Sundays for poor children in the area, and was also the base for Barnardo's evangelical missionary work. Activities at Hope Place soon grew to include weekly services for children, Bible classes for men, women and children, mothers' meetings, girls' sewing classes and a special service each weekday evening which was attended by an average of 130 boys. Plans were also being developed for a day school and a self-financing 'refuge' or hostel for orphan working boys who would pay three shillings a week for board and lodging.

At around this time, Barnardo encountered a destitute boy named Jim Jarvis who was to have a profound effect on his work. Jarvis, a homeless orphan, revealed how he and hundreds of boys like him slept rough in London each night. He led Barnardo through the backstreets of the area, and the two eventually climbed up onto the roof of an iron shed where eleven boys, dressed in rags and without covering of any kind, lay sleeping.

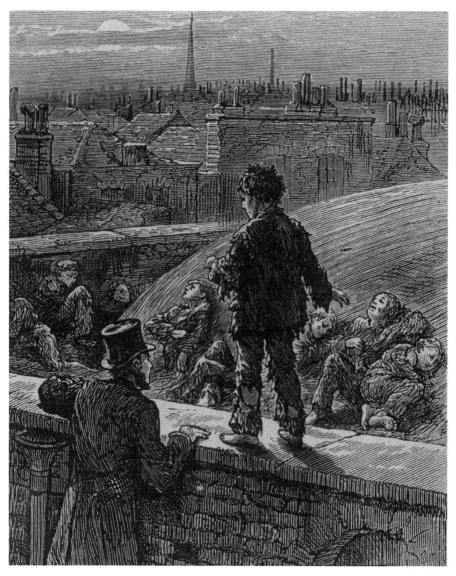

Jim Jarvis shows Barnardo homeless boys sleeping on a London rooftop.

Stepney Causeway

The plight of destitute children such as Jim Jarvis led Barnardo, in September 1870, to open his home for working lads at 18–20 Stepney Causeway. A couple of years later, the death of another homeless boy named John Somers – better known to his acquaintances as 'Carrots' because of his red hair – made a lasting impression on Barnardo.

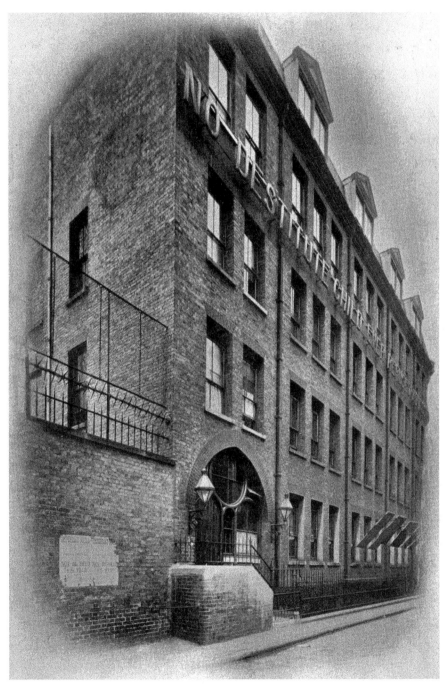

Barnardo's home for boys at Stepney Causeway, in the East End of London. Its famous slogan runs across the front of the building.

Lack of space at the Stepney Causeway home had resulted in 'Carrots' being denied admission and, a few nights later, he had been found dead from exposure and hunger. Barnardo was determined that such a thing should never happen again and in 1874 he opened 10 Stepney Causeway as the first of his open-all-hours shelters – later named Ever Open Door homes – whose boldly stated principle was 'No Destitute Child Ever Refused Admission'.

By the 1880s, Stepney Causeway was described as 'a large industrial voluntary home, providing maintenance, education and practical instruction in technical handicrafts to boys over 13 years of age'.[2] The premises also housed the administrative headquarters for the thirty-four institutions by then being run by Barnardo's organization.

In 1888, extensions were made to the Stepney Causeway home including the provision of workshops for training the boys in trades such as tailoring, boot-making, carpentry, brush-making, engineering, blacksmithing, tin-smithing, mat-making, wheel-making and harness-making. Barnardo also started to create employment for the boys through the formation of rag-collecting, wood-chopping and shoeb-lack brigades.

In 1888, medical care for Barnardo's children was enhanced by the opening of Her Majesty's Hospital, a state-of-the-art facility, at 13–19 Stepney Causeway. In 1899, Barnardo's took over the running of the

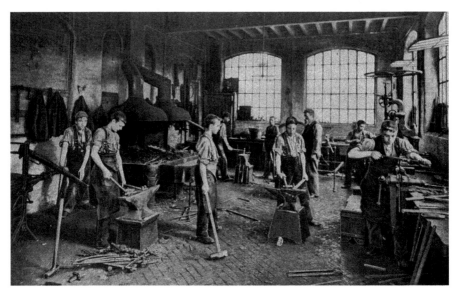

Boys at work in the blacksmith's shop at Stepney Causeway.

Marie Hilton Crèche at 12–16 Stepney Causeway. The Crèche, founded in 1871, provided day-care for the babies and children of working mothers and continued in operation until 1939.

Despite all the developments at Stepney Causeway, it was far from being the sole focus of Barnardo's activities. In 1872, his mission work moved to a new base in the Edinburgh Castle – a former gin palace and music hall in Limehouse which Barnardo converted into a working man's 'coffee palace' and People's Church. Three years later, he set up a large ragged school a few hundred yards away at Copperfield Road.

The Girls' Village Home

In June 1873, Barnardo, now aged 28, married Syrie Elmslie, two years his junior and the daughter of a city businessman. The couple had met when Syrie, who ran a ragged school in Richmond, invited Barnardo to speak at a meeting and entertainment event for poor boys.

As a wedding gift, the Barnardos were given the lease of Mossford Lodge, a large house in Barkingside near Ilford in Essex. Here, in the property's coach house, Barnardo was able to set up his first home for destitute and homeless girls, who were given training for domestic service. The home was managed by Syrie but she proved unsuited to the role. Barnardo also concluded that the girls needed a different style of accommodation.

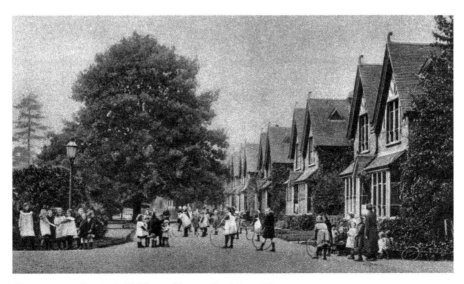

Playtime at the Girls' Village Home, Barkingside.

He began laying plans for a 'cottage homes' development on a plot of land adjacent to Mossford Lodge. This type of accommodation, which had originated on the continent, was just starting to be adopted in Britain, for example at the Farningham Home for Little Boys in Kent. Unlike the large buildings traditionally used as children's homes, cottage homes aimed to provide a more domestic scale of accommodation, with a village-like arrangement of houses set around a green. The children lived in small family-style groups, each household under the supervision of a house-mother. Fund-raising efforts for the scheme eventually allowed the first thirteen cottages of the Girls' Village Home to be opened in July 1876.

The Village Home eventually grew to include more than sixty cottages, housing around 1,500 girls. The site also included the Home's own schools, library, church, hospital and laundry.

Conflict and Controversy

The mid-1870s were a difficult time for Barnardo, triggered largely by the rivalry that had developed between various East End church missions. In 1874, a Baptist preacher named George Reynolds, who believed that many of his flock had been lured away by Barnardo's nearby Edinburgh Castle mission, began spreading false rumours about an improper relationship between Barnardo and a former landlady. In the same year, Fred Charrington – a member of the brewing family but with evangelical ambitions in his home area of Mile End – was angered by Barnardo's plans to open another large coffee palace and mission on Mile End Road to be known as the Dublin Castle. Reynolds and Charrington soon joined forces to mount a campaign against Barnardo through letters to the press which questioned his right to use the title 'Doctor', whether funds donated for his work were properly being accounted for, and reiterating the charge of sexual impropriety.

In light of the cost and publicity that would result from court proceedings, Barnardo was persuaded to refrain from legal action in return for a written promise from Reynolds and Charrington to end the matter. The question of his medical qualification did not go away, however, and he was embarrassed when a letter he produced from the University of Giessen concerning its award to him of an MD degree was shown to be a forgery. However, in the spring of 1876 he rectified matters by gaining a diploma at the Royal College of Surgeons in Edinburgh.

Further problems began at the end of 1876 when Reynolds published a pamphlet entitled *Startling Revelations* which claimed that Barnardo's homes were incompetently managed; that the children were mistreated, not given moral and religious instruction, and detained against their will; that Barnardo took money under false pretences and that he made misleading use of children's photos in his appeals. Fortuitously, over the previous year, Barnardo had been persuaded to place the ownership and legal responsibility for the homes in the hands of a board of trustees, served by a treasurer, an independent auditor, and with himself as lifetime honorary Director. After satisfying themselves that the accounts were in order, the trustees decided that the dispute should be submitted to a process of legal arbitration.

Barnardo emerged from the hearing relatively unscathed. The arbitrators found no evidence of financial malpractice or cruelty to children although they did criticize his former practice of placing miscreant boys in solitary confinement. Barnardo's resort to 'artistic fiction'

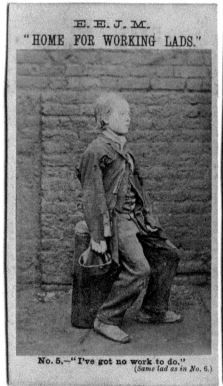
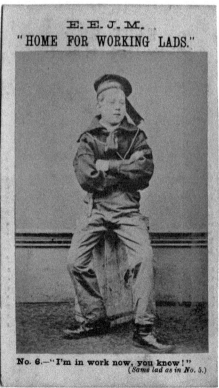

Barnardo's 'before-and-after' publicity pictures.

in his use of children's photos in his promotional materials was also censured, however. In conclusion, though, the arbitrators praised the valuable work being performed by Barnardo's homes which they saw as worthy of public confidence and support.

Barnardo's Goes National

Prior to the 1890s, Barnardo homes were almost exclusively located in and around London, with odd exceptions such as the one on Jersey, in the Channel Islands, a property which had been donated to the organization.

This changed in 1892 with the opening of seven Ever Open Door shelters in Bath, Cardiff, Edinburgh, Leeds, Liverpool, Newcastle upon Tyne and Plymouth. Over the next ten years, a similar number were gradually opened in other major centres such as Bristol, Birmingham and Belfast. The Edinburgh home was fairly short-lived – Barnardo's explicit policy of proselytizing all his children into the Protestant faith made the home's presence in the city less than welcome in Roman Catholic quarters.

As well as the Ever Open Doors, a number of provincial branch homes were gradually established including those in Exeter (1894), Epsom (1896), Cambridge (1897), Stockton-on-Tees (1899), Northampton (1902), Southampton (1902), Swansea (1902), Fakenham (1903) and Middlesbrough (1903).

In addition to these general homes, others were set up to provide particular forms of care. These included the Labour House, East London (1882, boys aged 17+), Babies' Castle, Hawkhurst, Kent (1884, babies and the under-6s), Felixstowe seaside home (1886, convalescents), Sheppard House, Bow (1887, physically disabled boys), the 'Beehive', Hackney (1889, girls' rescue/training home), the Jones Memorial Home, Southport (1894, physically disabled children), Home for Incurables, Bradford (1898, physically disabled children) and the Mare Street Home, Hackney (1900, deaf, dumb or blind children). In 1902, the opening of the Watts Naval Training School in Dereham in Norfolk remedied Barnardo's long-held desire to operate a boys' naval training ship.

In 1899, Barnardo's growing organization changed its formal legal status and became incorporated under the terms of the Companies Act of 1890, something that reduced the personal liability of the trustees. Its full name then became 'The National Incorporated Association for the Reclamation of Destitute Waifs, Otherwise Known as Dr Barnardo's Homes' but was still generally known simply as Dr Barnardo's Homes.

Emigration

As Thomas Barnardo was acutely aware, an 'ever-open door' to his homes could only be possible if there was an ever-open exit through which children could pass. For those who crossed his threshold, efforts were first made to find them accommodation with their relatives or friends. Children having particular religious affiliations, such as Roman Catholics, might be passed on for assistance from within their own faith community. For those who remained, then apart from long-term accommodation in his own homes, the two main options for 'disposal', as it was usually termed, were emigration and boarding out.

During the 1870s, Barnardo used the services of an independent emigration organizer, Miss Annie Macpherson, with around 500 of his children being migrated. The very first of these was none other than Jim Jarvis, Barnardo's first homeless boy, who went on to make a successful life for himself. South Africa and Canada were the main destinations. In some cases, emigration was used to benefit the health of particularly delicate children, but could also be provoked by the 'threatened interference of criminal or vicious relatives'.[3]

In 1882, Barnardo decided to set up his own emigration scheme, with an initial party of boys travelling to Ontario in August of that year under the supervision of the Governor of the Stepney Causeway Home, Frederick Fiedler. The first party of girls followed in July 1883 and in November of that year, Hazelbrae, a girls' distributing home, was opened in Peterborough, Ontario. The following year, Barnardo visited Canada to see the country for himself and also to reassure those he met that any children being sent there would be healthy, of good character and have received training in religious, moral and practical matters. In 1885, a Canadian headquarters was established at 214 Farley Avenue, Toronto, which also acted as a home for younger boys. In 1888, a 9,000-acre industrial farm was acquired near Russell, in the Shell River District of Manitoba, where older boys would initially be accommodated. In 1895, a further distributing home for younger boys was added in the west at 115 Pacific Avenue, Winnipeg.

Periodic concerns emerged about the welfare, treatment and monitoring of children sent to Canada but none proved serious enough to halt the traffic, with as many as a thousand Barnardo children making the passage each year up to 1915. A rosy image of the prospects that awaited young emigrants was presented in publicity photos published by the charity.

The First World War put emigration on hold but it resumed in 1920. In 1925, however, the Canadian government introduced a ban on the entry of parentless children under the age of fourteen. Small numbers of older Barnardo children continued to go there up until 1939.

A new destination for Barnardo's emigrants materialized after the First World War when Australia began a drive to expand its population – particularly with white settlers. The first party of forty-seven Barnardo boys travelled to the country in 1921, with the first consignment of girls arriving in 1923.

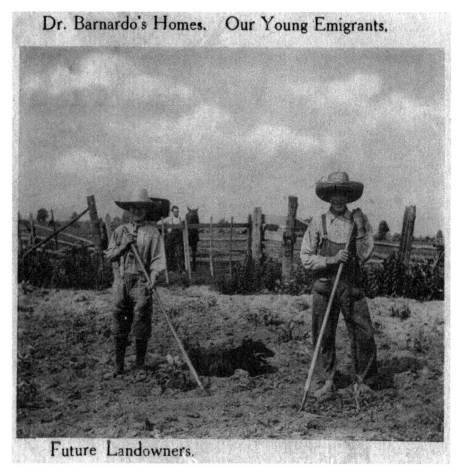

Barnardo's portrayal of what lay in store for its young emigrants.

The children were placed in homes and on farms in New South Wales and, from 1923, at the new Fairbridge Farm School in Pinjarra, near Perth in Western Australia. Fairbridge, named after its founder, Kingsley Fairbridge, provided training for younger children from under-privileged backgrounds. As at the Girls' Village Home, the children lived in family groups in cottages. By 1929, Barnardo's had set up its own farm school in Mowbray Park, Picton, but also continued to make use of Fairbridge.

The usual fate of the girls in Australia was domestic service but strict regulations were applied to their welfare. They were settled in groups, never in isolated locations, with a minimum weekly wage of fourteen shillings for those aged fourteen. Local Ladies' Committees were set up to visit and report on each girl's progress.

Numbers going to Australia slowed during the depression of the 1930s, with the country's government placing a bar on the immigration of boys over school age from 1931. At the end of 1938, the last pre-war party of Barnardo children set off for Australia, bringing the number sent since 1921 to the fairly modest total of 2,340. After the war, the scheme was resumed, finally ending in 1967.

Boarding Out

Boarding out, or what we would now usually refer to as fostering, had its origins in Scotland but by the 1880s was becoming more widely used by organizations involved in child care such as workhouse authorities. In 1887, Thomas Barnardo – recognizing the benefits of boarding out both for the children themselves and for relieving the pressure on places in his homes – placed 330 boys with 120 families in rural districts. Those he chose for boarding out were the younger ones, aged 5 to 9, who he felt suffered most from institutional care. The scheme was also limited to 'orphans', although this was a term he interpreted rather broadly as having one or both parents dead, or with both parents being deemed unsuitable.

The foster parents, all working class, were given a payment of five shillings a week for each child. They were required to have adequate accommodation that offered 'satisfactory sanitary conditions, pure moral surroundings, and a loving and Christian influence'.[4] They also had to sign a lengthy and detailed agreement as to how the children were to be treated. Regular inspection of the children was originally carried out by a specially employed female physician, with nurses later taking on the role.

The experiment proved a success, with the children settling in well and, with a very few exceptions, receiving satisfactory reports with regard to their health and educational progress. As a result, the scheme was expanded and, by 1892, more than 2,000 Barnardo children were being boarded out. Financial problems within the organization led to a fall in numbers in the 1890s, but by the time of Barnardo's death in 1905, over 4,000 children were being fostered, about a quarter of those being in Canada. One of the few complaints about the system was that on reaching the age of 14, children had to move back to one of the central homes to receive industrial or domestic training.

In 1889, Barnardo set up a pioneering scheme to board out illegitimate babies near to where their mothers were working. The unwed mother, who must have proved herself respectable and hard-working since her one mistake, was required to enter domestic service with an approved employer and could visit her child on her weekly half-day off. The mother shared the cost of the child's boarding out and the employer also received a payment from Barnardo's. If the mother failed to make her payment, the arrangement would be terminated and the child would go to an institutional home.

Barnardo Exits

Thomas Barnardo died on Tuesday, 19 September 1905, after suffering a series of angina attacks. He was 60 years old. Because of the enormous public interest in the event, special arrangements were made for the funeral. Barnardo's body lay in state at the Edinburgh Castle from Sunday 24 September until the morning of Wednesday 26th. A procession which included the staff and children from the homes and members of the organization's governing Council followed the coffin as it was taken through London's East End to Liverpool Street Station. The coffin travelled by a special train to Barkingside station and thence processed to the Girls' Village Home where the funeral service took place in a huge marquee erected on one of the greens. Afterwards, the coffin rested in the Home's church. A few days later, Barnardo's cremated remains were interred in the grounds.

New Boys' Homes

Although Barnardo had opened his Girls' Village Home in 1876, it was not until 1909 – four years after his death – that a comparable

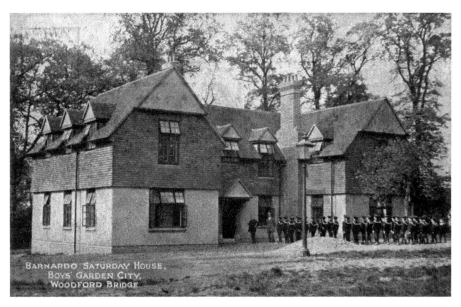

BARNARDO SATURDAY HOUSE,
BOYS' GARDEN CITY,
WOODFORD BRIDGE

Boys in naval uniform lined up outside the 'Barnardo Saturday' House at the Boys' Garden City.

establishment for boys began life. The Boys' Garden City, as the new home was named, was built at Woodford Bridge in Essex with much of the construction labour force being supplied by boys from the Stepney Boys' Home and Labour House. As with the Girls' Village, Woodford Bridge adopted the cottage homes principle with the boys living in family-style groups, each under the supervision of a resident house-mother. The Garden City was officially opened in 1912 and eventually accommodated around 700 boys, about half the number housed in the Girl's Village Home.

In 1919, The Russell-Cotes Sea Training School was opened at Parkstone in Dorset to train boys aged 13 to 16 for entry into the Merchant Navy. In 1922, the ageing industrial training facilities at Stepney Causeway were replaced by the William Baker Technical School, located on a country estate called Goldings near Hertford.

Wartime

The First World War (1914–18) had relatively little impact on Barnardo's activities although the contribution of its boys to the ranks of the fighting forces was much promoted.

World War Two was to prove rather different, however. As early as September 1938, the Home Office advised Barnardo's to move children from the Girls' Village Home and Boys' Garden City to safer locations in the south-west of England. Within three days, over 2,000 children had been evacuated.

With the declaration of war in September 1939, far more extensive plans were put into place for the evacuation of children from homes considered potentially vulnerable to enemy bombing. The government had urged owners of large country houses to make them available for wartime use and dozens of these were eventually occupied as Barnardo's evacuation centres, many located in East Anglia and in Scotland. Although such mansions might be viewed as the height of luxury, their new young residents were often crammed into back rooms with poor or non-existent plumbing. Water for washing had to be drawn in buckets from wells and the children bathed in kitchen sinks or tin baths in front of a fire. Local schools were unable to cope with such large influxes and the education of the evacuees often suffered as a result.

The 1940s also brought many changes behind the scenes at Barnardo's. Between the wars, steady improvements in state welfare

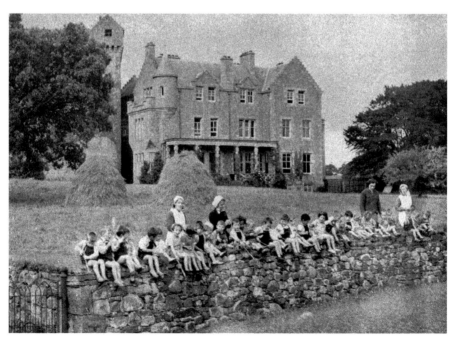

Barnardo evacuees during the Second World War at Comlongon Castle, Dumfries.

provision such as unemployment and sickness benefit, school meals and milk, and a schools' medical service, had made significant inroads into child poverty. The needs of deprived children were increasingly as much about the emotional and psychological as well as the physical. The war had also brought about an increased need for co-operation rather than competition with government departments, local authorities and other voluntary agencies. Pressure for a more modern and professional approach by the organization was highlighted by a Ministry of Health report about failings at Dame Margaret's, a Barnardo home in County Durham, where an 18-year-old girl was alleged to have been made pregnant by one of the boys.[5] Another challenge taken on by Barnardo's at this time was the running of two Approved Schools – Druids Heath in 1940, and the Quinta School, near Oswestry, in 1941.

To help meet these new demands, a staff training school was opened in Woodford Bridge in October 1941, with students studying topics such as the care and welfare of children, child psychology, first aid, hygiene, children's games, biblical story-telling, account-keeping, cookery and mending.

The Barnardo Rule Book

In 1944, as an adjunct to the new training programme, a confidential staff handbook was produced, providing detailed directions on every aspect of life in the homes. The 'Barnardo Book' included sections on such matters as the daily routine, health, maintenance of discipline, and sex education. Recommendations in the book included:

- training children from an early age to be useful about the house
- avoiding the imposition of silence at mealtimes as it savoured of 'Institution' rather than 'Home'
- training children in good table manners, the use of cutlery and looking after each other's wants
- punishing anyone talking in their dormitory after 'lights-out' by an early bedtime the following day
- sending enuresis cases to the lavatory at 10 p.m.
- limiting visits by parents or relatives to once a quarter
- inspecting all letters written or received by the children
- giving children weekly pocket money from the age of five.[6]

The Curtis Report

At the end of the Second World War, Barnardo's was at a low ebb. With the Girls' Village still requisitioned and evacuees being returned from their wartime foster-homes, the organization was struggling to find places for all the children being sent to it – it could no longer live up to its long-held promise, 'No destitute child ever refused admission'. The organization was also short of staff, and the wages it offered did not match those of other employers. And despite its efforts to update itself, Barnardo's image appeared increasingly old-fashioned.

An enormous challenge to the organization came in the shape of the Curtis Report, published in 1946, which favoured adoption as the best option for children lacking parents or a satisfactory home, with fostering the next best option, and institutional care as the least preferred alternative. Wherever possible, children were to maintain contact with relatives, and brothers and sisters kept together.

Although legal adoption had been possible since 1926, it was not something for which Barnardo's had shown much interest, still seeing itself as providing the substitute family for those that came into its care. Nonetheless, in 1947, Barnardo's became a registered adoption society. Under the 1948 Children Act, local authorities were required to set up a Children's Committee and appoint a Children's Officer to promote the welfare of deprived children. Instead of acting autonomously, charities such as Barnardo's now had to take their place in a national system of child care under the ultimate authority of the Home Office Children's Department.

Other changes came in the wake of the Curtis Report. There was a reduction in the amount of time that children in the homes spent doing household chores. The long-held notion that domestic service was the natural destination for Barnardo girls was also forced to change. There was a move towards making all the homes mixed, starting with the main sites in Barkingside, now renamed the Children's Village Home, and in Woodford Bridge, which became the Children's Garden City. Barnardo's administration, based in what was viewed as the hallowed ground of Stepney Causeway, was proving increasingly antiquated and inefficient and much of the charity's property was ageing and dilapidated.

The End of the Homes

In the 1950s and early 1960s, Barnardo's made significant progress in taking on board the evolving trends in providing care for disadvantaged children. In fact, by the mid-1960s, less than half of the 8,000 or so children in its care actually lived in the homes that it operated. The greater proportion were living, with various forms of Barnardo's support, with their own mothers, or with relatives or foster parents. However, many of the charity's staff and supporters still viewed the running of traditional children's homes as being its fundamental core activity. Despite the recommendations of the Curtis Report, the new homes opened by Barnardo's during this period were often still in large houses set apart from their local communities, such as Hatherley Brake near Cheltenham (1950), Elizabeth Bishop House in Warwick (1957) and Tudor Bank in Birkdale (1958). This was often in stark contrast to the activities of local councils who had taken over the responsibilities of the Poor Law authorities in 1930, including their often extensive provisions for pauper children. The growing numbers of children's homes provided by councils were now far more likely to be along modern lines – small in size and integrated into their local neighbourhoods.

A new course for Barnardo's was set in 1965 by its recently appointed General Superintendent, Mr V. L. Cornish. He proposed that, in light of the substantial provision of children's accommodation now being made by many local authorities, the charity should run down its own branch homes and direct more of its resources into new areas where the needs of children were not yet being met. In addition to adoption and fostering, these could include more specialized work with groups such as the physically handicapped, intellectually impaired, emotionally disturbed and behaviourally maladjusted.

This change in emphasis was marked, in January 1966, by a change in the organization's name from 'Dr Barnardo's Homes' to just 'Dr Barnardo's', shortened again in 1988 to 'Barnardo's'. Another significant event was the charity's momentous decision to leave its historic base at Stepney Causeway and relocate its administrative headquarters to a purpose-built office block at the Village Home site in Barkingside.

Despite much internal resistance and wrangling within Barnardo's, the increasing weight of professional opinion against residential care made change inevitable. Accordingly, the winding down of Barnardo's traditional homes went ahead with around ninety being closed between 1969 and 1980, the last going in 1989. Barnardo's change in emphasis was also indirectly aided by the 1970 Local Authority Social Services Act which led to council Children's Departments being subsumed under new social services departments. The change resulted in many former local authority staff with child care expertise being recruited by organizations such as Barnardo's.

From the 1970s onwards, Barnardo's continued to develop its work in areas such as adoption and fostering, the provision of family support centres especially in deprived areas such as inner cities, working with young offenders, and the growing concerns relating to children affected by sexual abuse and HIV/AIDS. Its work continues today, with more than 400 services currently being run across the UK providing support for children and families.

Chapter 8

The National Children's Home

Close on the heels of Barnardo was Thomas Bowman Stephenson, the founding father of what for much of its history was known as the National Children's Home (NCH) – now Action for Children. Stephenson was born in Newcastle upon Tyne on 22 December 1839, the seventh child of a Wesleyan Methodist minister and preacher, John Stephenson, and his wife Mary (née Bowman). His father's profession also meant that the family were moved around between a number of Methodist church circuits including Bedford, Dudley and Sheffield. Thomas became a committed Christian while at school in Dudley. Later, at Wesley College in Sheffield, he developed a liking and talent for public speaking and preaching. Stephenson's initial thoughts about a career had been to study law and become a barrister. This changed, however, during a stay with his parents who had returned to Tyneside. He stood in for a local minister who was ill and the response to his preaching was such that he instead began to think about entering the ministry, formally offering himself as a candidate in 1858. A month after examinations had taken place in London, he was accepted for training and spent the next two years at a Methodist college in Richmond, Surrey.

Stephenson's initial placements as a minister were in Norwich, Manchester and Bolton. His work was characterized by a willingness to find new ways of reaching people who would normally not enter a church, such as holding meetings in a theatre, or programmes of recitations and music. Stephenson was an accomplished singer and would sing at any opportunity, whether in church or while preaching from a chair in the street.

In 1868, Stephenson and his wife Ellen, whom he had married in 1864, were moved again – this time to take over the Waterloo Road Chapel in Lambeth, one of London's poorest areas. Again, he readily used novel means to make contact with non-church-goers, erecting a platform outside the chapel for open-air meetings. Realizing that people would be more likely to stay and listen if they could sit down, he appealed to his Methodist friends for donations to buy 200 chairs for the purpose.

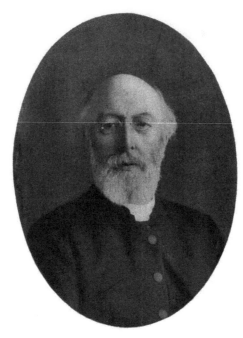

NCH founder Thomas Bowman Stephenson in about 1905.

One group that particularly came to Stephenson's attention in Lambeth were the numerous orphaned, abandoned and homeless children, many of whom were sickly and malnourished. He later wrote:

> *There they were, ragged, shoeless, filthy, their faces pinched with hunger, and premature wretchedness staring out of their too bright eyes, and I began to feel that now my time had come. Here were my poor little brothers and sisters sold to Hunger and the Devil, and I could not be free of their blood if I did not at least try to save some of them.*[1]

The First Homes

In March 1869, Stephenson, then aged 30, was approached by two fellow Methodists, Alfred Mager and Francis Horner, seeking his support for a fund-raising appeal they were launching. Mager, aged 32 and a banker by profession, and Horner, ten years his younger and a rising businessmen, were both involved in the running of the Sunday School at Lambeth's Clifton Street chapel. The two friends had also been conducting services in the notoriously rough Mint district of Southwark and their proposal was to open a model lodging house there to help down-and-out men. Stephenson, however, brought them round to the idea of a home for homeless and friendless boys, where training would also be provided. The plan was adopted and a small house found to rent at 8 Church Street (now Exton Street), Lambeth. Its very basic facilities included a dining room in a stable at the rear, and a loft that served as a dormitory. The 'training' consisted of chopping firewood.

The first two boys were received into the home on Friday, 9 July 1869. From the start, Stephenson – influenced by institutions such as the Rauhe House in Germany and the Mettray colony in France – wanted the home to be family-like in nature. The home was supervised by the resident 'house-parents', a Mr and Mrs Austin, whom the boys were expected to call 'Father' and 'Mother'.

On 16 July, a meeting was held at the home to promote the work. At the meeting, a formal constitution was agreed for the operation of The Children's Home, as the establishment was now called, which also included 'Instructions and Advice' for house-parents. A governing committee was appointed consisting of Mager and Horner, together with the Reverend C. H. Kelly and Mr W. T. Whelpton. Stephenson was appointed as the Home's Honorary Director.

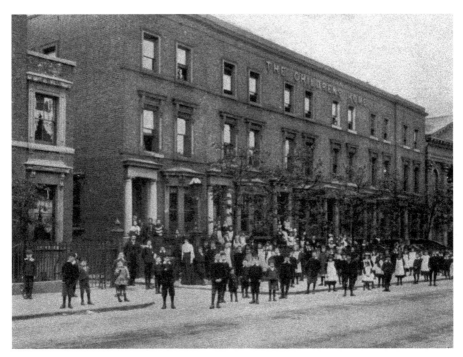

Inmates gathered outside the National Children's Home, Bonner Road, Bethnal Green.

Two months after its opening, the number of boys at Church Street had risen to more than twenty and an adjacent house was rented. Following Stephenson's transfer to the Bethnal Green circuit in 1871, it was decided that the home should be relocated to larger premises which were closer to his new location. The move, to 84 Bonner Road, Bethnal Green, took place in June 1871.

The new premises comprised a row of terraced houses along Bonner Road, plus a collection of buildings at the rear around a former stone-yard. Continuing Stephenson's ideal of a family-style structure, the children's accommodation was divided up into a number of single-sex households, with girls now being admitted for the first time.

Instead of the wood-chopping that had occupied the boys at Church Street, Bonner Road allowed a wider variety of industrial training to be provided, including baking, carpentry, plumbing and shoemaking. The printing department provided another training opportunity as well as producing a wide range of printed materials.

Over the following decades, the buildings were modified and extended, with the number of children accommodated eventually reaching more than three hundred.

Edgworth

In 1871, the donation of seventy acres of remote Lancashire moorland, complete with a public house, led to the creation of the Edgworth home, where country air and manual labour were viewed as the ideal remedy for children brought up in the squalor of East London. One of the Children's Home founders, city banker Alfred Mager, was the seemingly unlikely choice to go and manage the project but he was to continue as governor of Edgworth until his retirement in 1907.

The first arrivals at Edgworth were greeted by 'dirt and desolation; barren bog and dreary moss, stretching out before our gaw'.[2] They slept on straw and all hot water for cooking and washing had to be boiled on a small 'American stove'. During the Magers' first absence, the boys mutinied and went on the rampage. Mr Mager was alerted and returned at once. The boys were locked out and in the evening, when a thunderstorm broke, begged to be admitted. The ringleaders were thrashed and all thoughts of rebellion subdued.

Much of the early work needed was the construction of roads and drains and roadways. In later years, a reservoir was constructed to provide a reliable water supply for the home. The stone for construction work was extracted by the boys themselves from a local quarry east of the home.

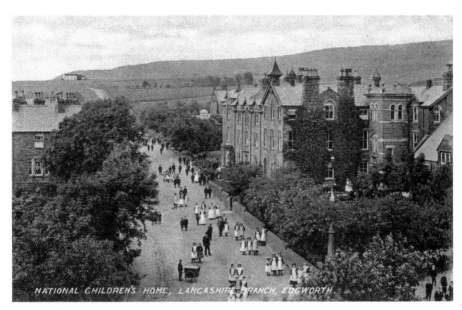

NATIONAL CHILDREN'S HOME, LANCASHIRE BRANCH, EDGWORTH.

A bird's-eye view of the NCH 'Home on the Moors' in Edgworth.

The children's accommodation was organized as family-group homes each with around sixteen boys or girls under the supervision of a 'sister'. Many of the houses were named after those whose donations had financed their construction. There were eventually around twenty houses, accommodating a total of over 300 children. The site also had its own school, hospital, swimming bath, workshops, bakery, dairy and farm.

Further Expansion

A succession of other homes followed. An Industrial School was opened in 1875 in Milton, near Gravesend in Kent. The School housed up to 160 boys aged from 8 to 14 years, most placed there by the courts.

In 1880, an existing children's home was taken over in Ramsey on the Isle of Man, following the death of its founder. Two years later, the Princess Alice Orphanage in Sutton Coldfield, near Birmingham, was a purpose-built 'cottage homes' development, eventually housing around 300 children. The main donor's stipulation that it be only for orphans made it the only NCH home to have the word 'orphanage' in its name, and resulted in the charity becoming officially known as The Children's Home and Orphanage.

Special care for convalescent children was introduced with the opening of the Alverstoke home in 1887. Further provision for convalescent and physically disabled children came with the Chipping Norton home in 1903.

The years leading up the First World War marked a major surge in growth, with large cottage home sites being established in Frodsham in Cheshire (1903), in Bramhope near Leeds (1906) and in Harpenden in Hertfordshire (1913), the latter also becoming the headquarters branch of what from 1908 was officially known as the National Children's Home and Orphanage. A TB (tuberculosis) sanatorium was opened near the Harpenden home site in 1910 and, in the same year, an existing home in Cardiff was taken over to become the charity's first property in Wales.

Following Stephenson's retirement in 1900, he was succeeded as Director by Arthur Gregory. Gregory held the post until his sudden death in 1912, the same year that Stephenson died.

The First World War had little impact on the Home and the number of branches doubled between 1909 and 1929. Over the same period, the number of children being cared for rose by 75 per cent.

Staff Training

From an early stage in the development of the NCH, the importance of staff training was recognized. In March 1873, the Home's Committee

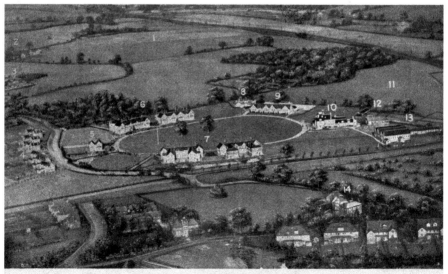

1. Farm of 260 acres. 2. Farm House and Buildings. 3. Sanatorium 4. Staff Houses. 5. Governor's House. 6. Girls' Houses. 7. Boys' Houses. 8. Laundry. 9. Schools. 10. Administration Block. 11. Playing Fields. 12. Chapel. 13. Workshops for Trade Training. 14. Apprentices' Hostel.

An aerial view of the NCH cottage homes site in Harpenden, identifying the various sections.

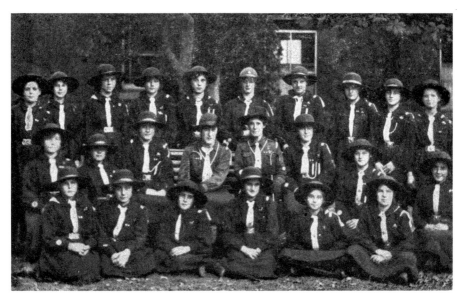

Girl Guides at the NCH home in Alverstoke, Hampshire. Following the founding of the movement in 1910, many girls' homes established their own Guide
Companies.

noted that two men and one woman had 'offered themselves to assist
in the work of the Home, with a view to being trained for Christian
labour, and have been accepted by the House Committee'.[3]

By the end of the 1870s, the joint recruitment of men and women was
abandoned and a scheme was begun to train 'Sisters of the Children'
who would look after the 'family groups' around which the homes
were organized. At the outset, a number of 'old girls' of the Home
were made into Probationer Sisters. Their training day included helping with the domestic work until 10 a.m., exercise such as a walk in the
park from 10 to 11 a.m., then lessons until 1 p.m. given by 'an educated
lady' in a room allocated for the purpose.[4]

Soon after the new training scheme was established, Stephenson
began to appeal more widely for women with such a vocation to
become sisters. This could either be as Sisters of the Children (often
shortened to just 'Sisters') or, in a wider evangelical missionary role,
as Sisters of the People, or Deaconesses as they were more usually
known.

A contribution of £500 by a Mr William Mewburn enabled the
setting up of a sisters' training home, named Mewburn House, at 7
Agnes Terrace, later relocated to the Home's main site at 84 Bonner

Road. In 1898, Willard House, a property near the Bonner Road home, became a training establishment specifically for Sisters of the Children. It accommodated seven students who, as well as running the house themselves, learnt cooking, washing, the making of children's clothes, with studies in Bible knowledge, theology, and nursing. The trainees also spent time in the houses of the Children's Home and took charge when the sisters were ill or had an afternoon off.

In 1935, the sisters' training home moved to Stephenson Hall, a purpose-built facility at the NCH's administrative headquarters in Highbury Park, North London, and arguably the country's first child care training college. The syllabus at Stephenson Hall included Bible study, child study (psychology), child guidance (psychiatry), English, principles of social work, first aid and home nursing, nature study, housewifery, cookery and dressmaking. There was also recreational instruction such as toy-making, keep-fit classes, and a Girl Guide Cadet Corps.

In 1946, the Princess Alice College, an establishment specifically for the training of sisters, was opened at the Princess Alice Orphanage near Birmingham. It closed in 1960 and its function was taken over by Stephenson Hall.

For many of the women who became sisters, it was a lifetime's vocation. Some were also ordained Methodist ministers. By the 1970s, however, the numbers of women coming forward to join the sisterhood was in decline. For those wanting to work as child care professionals, a much wider range of opportunities now existed, for example in local authority Children's Departments, which often offered better salaries and more flexible career paths. The number of traditional homes being run by the NCH was also falling. It seemed inevitable that the sisterhood would eventually fold and in March 1985 a majority of the last eighteen serving sisters agreed to its closure.

Emigration

Like Barnardo's, the Children's Home faced the constant problem of making provision for the flow of children that came its way. Emigration to countries such as Canada played an important part in dealing with this problem, as well as being seen as giving children the opportunity of a better future than they might find in Britain. Canada had a special attraction for the Home's Principal, Thomas Stephenson, who viewed it as a particularly moral and egalitarian country.

In June 1872, Stephenson visited the USA and Canada where he met Dr Morley Punshon, a preacher and supporter of Stephenson's work, who accompanied him on the tour. In Hamilton, Ontario, he met Senator W. E. Sanford who subsequently became Treasurer of the Canadian branch. Support in Hamilton also materialized in the raising of £1,000 to buy a house and land to establish a distributing home.

The clearest message that Stephenson picked up on his visit was that Canada would embrace youngsters who were equipped with manual skills for their new life, whereas untrained children would not be welcome. If this condition were met, he was assured, then the only difficulty would be in supplying all the applicants requesting his children.

The scheme was given approval by the Methodist Conference and a property was acquired at 1078 Main Street, Hamilton. The first governor was a respected citizen of Winnipeg, Mr R. T. Riley.

In May 1873, the first party of thirty-four boys and fifteen girls sailed for Canada in the charge of Francis Horner, one of the Children's Home's co-founders. By September, Horner was able to report that 200 applications for the children had been received, and they had finally been placed with forty-five families of which thirty-seven belonged to the Wesleyan Methodist Church. Twenty-six of the boys had joined farming families, two were learning carpentry, two the blacksmith's and wheelwright's trades, two were employed in Senator Sanford's warehouse, and two were 'printer boys' in the Methodist Book-room in Toronto. Five of the girls had been adopted into Christian families, six had been taken on as domestic servants, and four had gone into farming families.

In 1874, Stephenson himself accompanied a party of ten boys and thirty girls to Canada. His report of the visit detailed the arrangements that had been put in place for the care and monitoring of the children:

> *The Children's Home in Hamilton is a pleasant place. There are about eight acres of good land, which produces grapes, peaches, and strawberries in profusion, as well as the plainer and more substantial vegetables. There is a well-built brick house, and a large wooden house behind, containing dormitory, dining room, and lavatory, intended for the reception of the young emigrants on their first arrival. The use of such a Canadian centre is threefold. It is a reception house for the children on their arrival in the country. It is also a house of shelter for any of them who, through sickness or other causes, are thrown out of the situations to which they are sent; and it is a residence and office for the governor or agent, who keeps up a frequent correspondence with the children, and visits them at regular intervals. In any good system of juvenile emigration there should certainly be supervision*

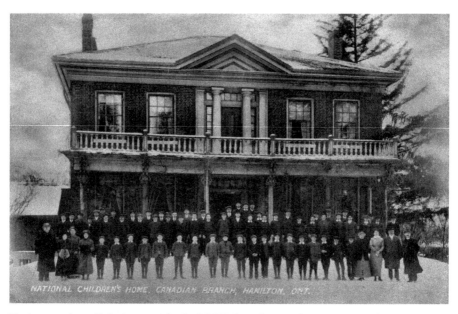

Emigrants from Britain outside the NCH distributing home in Hamilton, Ontario.

of the children, and a more or less authoritative guardianship over them for at least three years after their arrival in their adopted land.

When the time draws near at which a party of children is expected, a notice to that effect is inserted in one or two newspapers; and forthwith each mail brings in applications. To every applicant is sent a printed paper of questions; from the answers to which a judgement may be formed as to his status and character, and as to the sort of boy or girl he desires to have. This application must be accompanied by a certificate of character from a magistrate or clergyman, and preference is given to those who are members of some Christian communion. To the applicants the children are then allotted, after a careful consideration of each child's character and probable fitness for the situation.[5]

Despite occasional criticism of the treatment or monitoring that some children received in Canada, emigration soon became the fate of most of those leaving the Children's Home. By 1909, of the 3,709 of the children who had ever left the care of the Home, 2,157 (58 per cent) had gone to Canada, with 50 more to Australia and New Zealand.[6]

Emigration was halted during the First World War and, with increasing restrictions being imposed by the Canadian government, numbers declined sharply. From 1924, a complete bar was imposed on immigrants who were below working age. As a result, the Hamilton home finally closed in 1934.

With the ending of emigration to Canada, a new destination emerged in the shape of Australia. In the years up to the Second World War, a few groups of children had been sent to Australian institutions such as the Fairbridge Farm School. After the war, the Australian government launched a drive to promote immigration, including that of children, with financial support provided for their settlement. In 1947, it announced a target of 50,000 children, which were mainly being sought from Britain and Europe. Encouragement to make use of the scheme was given to NCH by the Northcote Farm School in Victoria, to which the NCH had sent thirty-three boys and four girls before the war.[7]

The NCH's then principal, John Litten, visited Australia in 1948 and was impressed by what he was told – the Australian government would not only pay the travel costs of children emigrating, but also give a grant towards the equipping any establishments set up by the Home. In addition, the existing Methodist Children's Home in Melbourne had offered to take up to fifty children aged from 4 to 10 years. Litten's proposal to canvass all the parents and guardians of the children in the care of the Home as to their interest in the scheme received a lukewarm reception, however. Some members of the charity's executive body and the then Principal Designate, John Waterhouse, felt that more caution was needed before the

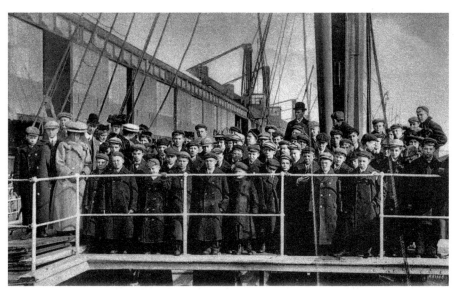

An NCH emigration party about to set sail for Canada, early 1900s.

Home committed itself too deeply. As a result, the numbers of the Home's children migrating to Australia were small, fifty-three boys and twenty-nine girls in the first year, but a total of only ninety-one over the whole of the period 1950–54. The children that did go underwent a month-long preparation at the Alverstoke home. They were settled at four locations: Dalmar, Carlingford, Sydney; Magill, Adelaide; Cheltenham, Melbourne and Victoria Park, Perth. A sister was sent to accompany each group.[8]

Some aspects of the scheme received criticism from the parents of children sent to Australia. Despite assurances that children unhappy in their new surroundings could be sent back, it transpired that this would only happen on a payment of £65 (a relatively large amount at that date) being made to cover the cost of the return passage. It also emerged that some children had been separated from the brothers and sisters they had previously lived with in children's homes back in Britain.

The Curtis Report

The Curtis Committee was established by the government in 1946 to review existing provision for children lacking a normal family home. Its membership included the NCH's John Litten. The Committee's report expressed the view that adoption and boarding out (fostering) were preferable to institutional care. If the latter was needed, then it should be in small homes, with children encouraged to maintain contact with relatives. Better staff training was also needed.

The NCH had been involved in boarding out on a modest scale since the 1880s. By the 1930s, however, only 7 per cent of its children were being placed in foster care and then only up until the age of 7 or 8 when they were recalled into institutional care at one of its homes. Following the introduction of legal adoption in 1926, it had also become an approved adoption agency, although by the late 1930s it was only processing around forty adoptions a year. As regards its own homes, the NCH had pioneered the training of staff and the 'family group' system was central to its philosophy. Despite the Curtis Committee's recommendations, the NCH still saw its primary role as providing residential care. This was something that was to take many years to change. One alteration that did take place, though, was the dropping of 'and Orphanage' from the charity's name.

The End of the Homes

Between 1950 and 1969, under the directorship of John Waterhouse, a gradual change began to take place in the direction of the charity. During that period, fourteen old homes were closed and eighteen new ones opened, although some of these such as Newcastle and Scarborough were simply relocations of existing branch homes. Others, such as two hostels in Manchester, the nursery in Ealing, and the Springside nursery and the Firbank diabetic unit (both in Frodsham) reflected a growing trend towards more targeted provision. This was also apparent in the eight homes that changed their use during this period, with the Edgworth and Bramhope becoming Special Schools, and the former Elmfield TB Sanatorium in Harpenden being converted to a Special School for physically handicapped children.

The tide was turning away from the Home's long-held principle of 'rescuing' children from bad surroundings and towards alternatives such as boarding out, adoption and supporting families to allow children to stay with their natural parents. Charities such as the NCH were increasingly affected by the financial burden of providing long-term residential care, and by the growing provision of residential care by local authorities. Enormous social changes also took place in the 1960s and '70s, such as the rise in the numbers of single-parent families, divorces and couples cohabiting. The children in need of new homes were increasingly likely to be older, have a disability, have emotional or social problems or be from an ethnic minority.

The 1980s onwards saw a major change in the NCH's focus towards more specialist projects. These included residential facilities for children with particular physical, mental or emotional difficulties, family support schemes, and help for young offenders, homeless youngsters and those leaving care.

As the organization re-orientated itself, the large old homes were gradually wound down and eventually sold off. Two of the biggest sites, Harpenden and Frodsham, both closed in 1985. The same year marked the disbanding of the sisterhood, the group of devoted women who for many years had managed the charity's homes.

In 1994, reflecting its new outlook, the charity was renamed NCH Action for Children with the name being shortened in 2008 to just Action for Children. Still working in partnership with the Methodist Church, the charity's hundreds of services currently include adoption and fostering, family support and the running of specialist schools.

Chapter 9

The Waifs and Strays Society

The final member – alongside Barnardo's and the NCH – of what is sometimes referred to as the 'Big Three', was the Waifs and Strays Society (now the Children's Society), founded in 1881 by Edward de Montjoie Rudolf. He was born on 11 April 1852, at 63 Pleasant Place, West Square, Lambeth. Edward was the second son of Major William Edward Rudolf, a 67-year-old former officer in the Light Dragoons and the Dutch Army, and his wife Susan, who was almost fifty years his junior. The family were relatively poor and neither Edward nor his younger brother, Robert, attended school but were taught by their father, a somewhat stern and authoritarian figure, with rigid religious beliefs. The Major, who was something of a linguist, earned a little money by translation work. As his eyesight grew increasingly poor, he was helped in the work by young Edward, whose upbringing was characterized by strictness, financial insecurity, religious observance and a sense of duty.[1]

At around the age of 14, he started work as an office boy in Blackfriars. He also studied in the evening to try and remedy his lack of formal education. His father then secured him a post as a junior clerk at the Dutch Consulate. Sometime in around 1868, Rudolf was walking home from work one evening when he came across a small boy sitting alone on a doorstep. The boy was homeless and had nowhere to go. Unsure what to do, Rudolf eventually found the boy shelter for the night at the local police station. The small incident planted a seed that was to set the direction of Rudolf's life. In September 1869, he became involved in the running of a Popular Educator Class held at the rear of Walworth Road Chapel. Six months later he decided that his life's ambitions were to enter the Ministry, and also to found an orphanage for outcast and destitute children.

Over the next decade, these ambitions slowly came to fruition. In 1870, Rudolf started studying Greek and Divinity at the City of London College. The following year, he passed the Civil Service examination and took up a post at the Office of Works, Whitehall. He opened a successful night school at St Philip's church in Kennington then, after the family moved to new lodgings at Portland Place, Kennington, became superintendent of the Sunday School in the parish of St Anne's, a post he held for ten years. He became increasingly involved in the work of the parish, while at the same time was steadily advancing his career up the Office of Works. He also found time, in 1874, to join the Guild of St Alban's, a brotherhood of devout laymen who assisted the clergy by undertaking social work in deprived urban areas. One of the brothers' duties was a devotion 'to the education of the young in the doctrine and discipline of the Church, to reclaiming the lost and raising the fallen'.[2] Another important event during this period was his encounter with the Bulmers, a fairly well-to-do family in the parish whose two daughters, Minnie and Emma, were considered local beauties. Emma, although having studied art in South Kensington, was employed as a painter at Doulton's pottery works. She was later to become a novelist, an inventor, a suffragette, and a member of the Fabian Society. At Rudolf's suggestion, Emma became a teacher at the St Anne's Sunday School. Before too long, a romance developed and the two became engaged in 1879.

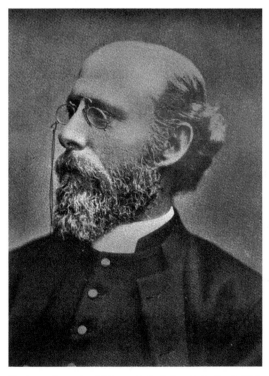

Waifs and Strays Society founder Edward de Montjoie Rudolf in about 1897.

The Founding of the Society

In 1880, two small boys who had been regular attendees at the Sunday School abruptly stopped coming. It transpired that, after the death of their father, their hard-pressed mother had been struggling to keep going rather than resort to the workhouse. After much searching to find the boys a home that did not require payment, they had eventually been taken by an 'Undenominational Home' – Barnardo's, in fact. The homes run by Thomas Barnardo gave their inmates an avowedly Protestant upbringing, but he aligned himself with no particular denomination or religious creed, something which caused suspicion among churchmen such as Edward Rudolf. More specifically, Rudolf felt he had betrayed the principle of the Guild of St Alban to educate the young in the doctrines of the Church of England, to which they would now be lost. It was clearly time for him to act.

Over the next year or so, Rudolf aired his ideas for establishing a 'Central Home for Waifs' to be run by the Anglican Church. Reactions were varied. Some described the scheme as 'crack-brained'. Others questioned the need for yet another society running homes in addition to those already provided by the Poor Law authorities, Dr Barnardo, the Methodist Children's Home, and hundreds of smaller charities. Maria Rye, a promoter of children's emigration to Canada, felt that girls should be the focus of any new home, as they faced particular problems and dangers. Many, however, unreservedly welcomed the idea and offered financial support. An important supporter of the scheme was a prosperous vinegar manufacturer named Mark Beaufoy. As well as making a donation of £50, Beaufoy offered the use of his imposing house for the formative meeting at Caron Place, South Lambeth, where, on 21 March 1881, the Church of England Children's Society was born.

The initial meeting formed a committee and agreed 'to establish a Central Home in connection with the Church of England for the reception of destitute children'. The Church of England in fact already operated a number of children's homes around the country, but these were not intended to provide emergency accommodation for the homeless or destitute. The aim of the envisaged Central Home – or rather Homes, one for boys and one for girls – was to receive and hold children until arrangements could be made for their placement and maintenance at one of the existing homes.

At their next meeting, the committee resolved that any homes that they set up should, as far as possible, provide children with a family environment rather than an institutional one. This is something that would distinguish the homes from the grand edifices established by many other organizations. It was also agreed that the patronage of the Archbishop of Canterbury, Dr Archibald Tait, should be sought. A deputation met the Archbishop on 27 June 1881 and, two months later, after careful consideration of the matter, he gave his support to the new Society. In the meantime, on 6 July 1881, Edward Rudolf and Emma Bulmer celebrated their marriage.

The Society's First Home

On 16 December 1881, after looking at a number of properties, the Society's committee decided to rent a small house at 8 Stamford Villas, Friern Road, East Dulwich where twelve girls could be accommodated. The home opened its doors early in 1882. With a long-standing civil servant like Edward Rudolf involved, it was inevitable that a comprehensive set of rules should be drawn up for the running of the home. These included:

- Children to rise in summer at 6.30, in winter at 7.00.
- On leaving the bedrooms, beds to be stripped, and windows thrown wide open top and bottom, unless it be either raining, snowing or foggy weather, in which case they must only be opened a little at the top.
- After prayers, breakfast at 7.30, in summer, and 8.00 in winter.
- After breakfast, girls above 9 to be set in turns, day about, to help the matron in the house, kitchen and laundry work; girls above 8 may help to make beds, wash up, and such light work.
- Dinner to be at 1.00 p.m.
- Children to attend school twice daily.
- Saturday being a holiday at school, all girls above 9 are to clean the house from top to bottom.
- Little ones to be in bed by 7 o'clock, those under 9 by 8 o'clock, under 12 by 8.30, above 12 by nine o'clock.
- Prayers, with a short portion of Scripture, to be read before breakfast and after tea.
- Tea to be at 5.30 in the winter, and at 6 in summer.
- Children to be taught a simple prayer (in addition to the Lord's Prayer) to be said at their bedsides morning and evening.
- The matron is to see that the children are washed to their waists, before going to bed; that they wash their face and hands in the morning, and that they are bathed once a week; also that their hair is cut short on their admission and kept perfectly clean.

They should wash it every morning when washing their faces and rub it perfectly dry.

- If the matron wishes for a day or two's holiday at any time, she must put her request before the local committee at the monthly meeting on the first Wednesday in the month.[3]

The mention of the local committee in the final item indicates Rudolf's clear philosophy that management of the homes was not to be controlled by the central organization, but largely devolved to a locally constituted body. This was another feature that distinguished the Society from other large children's organizations, although it later sometimes proved to be a source of problems.

Rudolf also devised a weekly dietary, or menu, plan, indicating how each child was to be fed on his suggested sum of 3s. 6d. a week:

Breakfast

- Sundays, bread and butter, with cocoa.
- Weekdays, porridge and milk, and bread; and bread and dripping, with milk and water, on alternate days.

Dinner

- Sunday, meat, vegetables, rice pudding, or stewed rhubarb, or fruit in summer.
- Monday, soup with thick round of bread and milk pudding, alternating with boiled apple or rhubarb pudding.
- Tuesday, Irish stew with rice and carrots, or a dripping crust.
- Wednesday, boiled suet pudding with treacle.
- Thursday, meat and green vegetables, with a little bread.
- Friday, soup and bread, and a milk pudding.
- Saturday, baked suet pudding with raisins, apples or carrots.

Supper

- Sundays, bread and butter, and tea.
- Weekdays, bread and dripping and bread and treacle alternating, with milk and water.[4]

The first girl to enter the Dulwich Home was Isabella Trotter-Williams, an illegitimate child whose mother, a Miss or Mrs Williams, had died when Isabella was three. She had then lived with a Mrs Trotter on Ratcliffe Highway. After Mrs Trotter died when Isabella was 14, the girl was taken into the Dulwich Home. It was then decided that Isabella

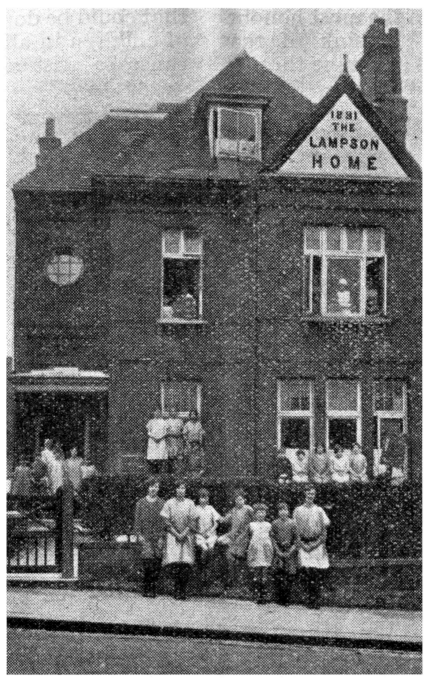

The first Waifs and Strays Society establishment – the Lampson Home, East Dulwich.

was an ideal candidate for emigration to Canada. She was accordingly dispatched to a home in Peckham run by Miss Rye who organized emigration parties of such children. The £10 fee (plus outfit) for the arrangement was paid by the Society. Isabella's outfit comprised:

> *'Outfit' Dress given her by a lady*
> *New flannel petticoat*
> *Chemise belonging to the house she came from. Marked*
> *Stockings she came in*
> *Old pair of boots given her by Miss Rye*
> *Hat she came in*
> *Old petticoat of her own*[5]

In 1884, the Dulwich Home moved to a larger property at 62 Overhill Road, originally called Baroda House but renamed the Lampson Home for Girls in 1887.

Expansion

In February 1882, soon after the original Dulwich home opened, a receiving home for boys was established at Aveley Road, Clapton. A third home, for girls, was opened in late 1882 at Old Quebec Street, Marylebone.

The response to the opening of these first homes soon made it apparent that, despite the provision already being made by other charities and by the Poor Law authorities, the problem of destitute and homeless children on the streets of the nation's towns and cities was enormous. In April 1883, the Society decided to establish boys' and girls' Receiving Homes in every Anglican diocese. Plans were already forming for a Receiving Home in Canada. All children's homes with Church of England affiliations were contacted as potential recipients of the children being received. Efforts were also being made, particularly in rural areas to find foster parents. By the end of the year, however, it had become apparent that in order to meet the demand it had opened up, the Society would itself need to operate long-term residential homes. Reflecting this, the Society changed its name from 'The Church of England Central Home for Waifs and Strays' to 'The Church of England Central Society for Providing Homes for Waifs and Strays' – usually shortened to just 'The Waifs and Strays Society'.

The homes expanded rapidly. In 1882, the Society had thirty-four children in its care; by 1902, this had risen to three thousand and seventy-one. Likewise, the number of its homes over the same period rose from two to ninety.[6]

From the outset, the Society used four different routes to find homes for the children it received. These were passing children on to other organizations, the use of boarding out, assisted immigration to Canada and placement in the Society's own homes. These channels varied in what children they could absorb, however. The Society restricted placements with foster parents to children under the age of seven. Emigration was limited by the Canadian authorities to children over twelve. And the total amount of accommodation provided by other organizations was relatively static. There was a particular need to find homes for children aged 10 or over.

Pressure for places in the Society's homes also came from the workhouse authorities who, since 1862, had been empowered to board out children in establishments run by other bodies and that had been approved for the purpose. The Society's ideal of 'saving' children from an institutional upbringing in the workhouse meant that it felt obliged to rise to this challenge.

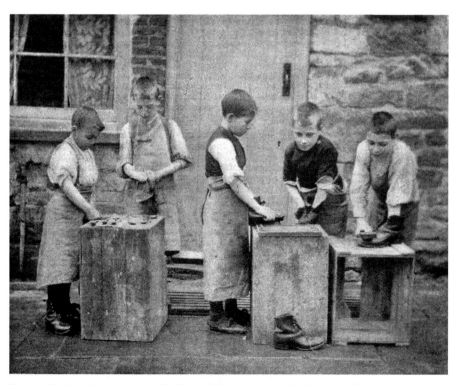

Boys polishing boots at the Waifs and Strays Society's Lincoln Home.

As the Society became established and well known, properties were increasingly donated to it. In some cases, such as the Stroud Green Home for Girls, these were existing children's homes which were in danger of closing for some reason – perhaps their finances were shaky, or their founders wished to retire. In other cases, properties were given to the Society which could be turned into a home, as happened in 1913 with Hatton Hall in Wellingborough, which became the Hatton Home for Boys.

Boarding Out

The Society's emphasis on placing children in a family environment made boarding out, or fostering, an attractive option. And so long as there was a good supply of suitable foster parents, it was potentially also more flexible in dealing with occasional surges in the demand for places than in trying to provide the accommodation in the Society's own homes.

The Society fostered its first child – Case No. 7, Jane Bellamy – in June 1883, with a family in Wiltshire. Over the next thirty years, around a quarter of the children in the Society's care were fostered each year. Wherever possible, homes were found in rural areas – as well as providing healthy surroundings, such locations were also less likely to receive unwelcome visits from a child's own parents.

Much of the groundwork in finding foster homes was placed in the hands of local clergy who, together with other suitable people from the area, also supervised the children and submitted reports on them every three months.

Boarded out children and their foster parents occasionally had group outings such as the annual summer treat provided by Mrs and Mrs George Willis in their garden at Claremont, Leighton Buzzard.

Despite supervision and regulations, cases of neglect or cruelty occasionally surfaced. In 1893, the Society appointed a professional inspectress who toured the country making unannounced visits to the Society's homes.

Emigration

In 1884, the Waifs and Strays Society decided to set up its own emigration scheme, following a similar move by Barnardo's two years earlier. The Society launched an appeal for £1,000 to fund the project and the target was soon reached, much aided by a donation of £250 from Mrs Henry Huck Gibbs. The Reverend John Bridger, a clergyman who

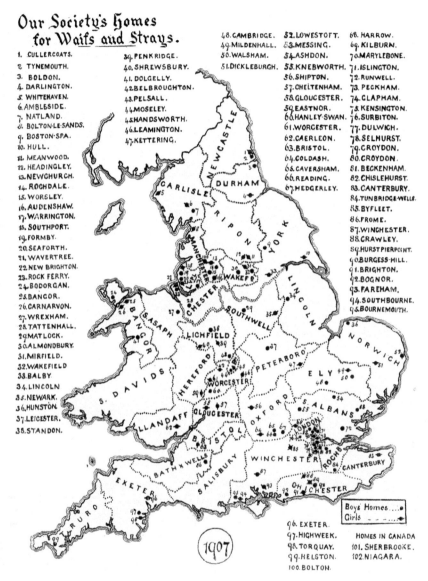

Our Society's Homes for Waifs and Strays.

1. CULLERCOATS.
2. TYNEMOUTH.
3. BOLDON.
4. DARLINGTON.
5. WHITEHAVEN.
6. AMBLESIDE.
7. NATLAND.
8. BOLTON-LE-SANDS.
9. BOSTON-SPA.
10. HULL.
11. MEANWOOD.
12. HEADINGLEY.
13. NEWCHURCH.
14. ROCHDALE.
15. WORSLEY.
16. AUDENSHAW.
17. WARRINGTON.
18. SOUTHPORT.
19. FORMBY.
20. SEAFORTH.
21. WAVERTREE.
22. NEW BRIGHTON.
23. ROCK FERRY.
24. BODORGAN.
25. BANGOR.
26. CARNARVON.
27. WREXHAM.
28. TATTENHALL.
29. MATLOCK.
30. ALMONDBURY.
31. MIRFIELD.
32. WAKEFIELD
33. BALBY.
34. LINCOLN
35. NEWARK.
36. HUNSTON.
37. LEICESTER.
38. STANDON.

39. PENKRIDGE.
40. SHREWSBURY.
41. DOLGELLY.
42. BELBROUGHTON.
43. PELSALL.
44. MOSELEY.
45. HANDSWORTH.
46. LEAMINGTON.
47. KETTERING.

48. CAMBRIDGE.
49. MILDENHALL.
50. WALSHAM.
51. DICKLEBURGH.
52. LOWESTOFT.
53. MESSING.
54. ASHDON.
55. KNEBWORTH.
56. SHIPTON.
57. CHELTENHAM.
58. GLOUCESTER.
59. EASTNOR.
60. HANLEY-SWAN.
61. WORCESTER.
62. CAERLEON.
63. BRISTOL.
64. COLDASH.
65. CAVERSHAM.
66. READING.
67. HEDGERLEY.

68. HARROW.
69. KILBURN.
70. MARYLEBONE.
71. ISLINGTON.
72. RUNWELL.
73. PECKHAM.
74. CLAPHAM.
75. KENSINGTON.
76. SURBITON.
77. DULWICH.
78. SELHURST.
79. CROYDON.
80. CROYDON.
81. BECKENHAM.
82. CHISLEHURST.
83. CANTERBURY.
84. TUNBRIDGE-WELLS.
85. BYFLEET.
86. FROME.
87. WINCHESTER.
88. CRAWLEY.
89. HURST PIERPOINT.
90. BURGESS-HILL.
91. BRIGHTON.
92. BOGNOR.
93. FAREHAM.
94. SOUTHBOURNE.
95. BOURNEMOUTH.

96. EXETER.
97. HIGHWEEK,
98. TORQUAY,
99. HELSTON.
100. BOLTON.

HOMES IN CANADA
101. SHERBROOKE.
102. NIAGARA.

Boys' Homes .....•
Girls — — — — —

1907

A 1907 map showing the locations of the Waifs and Strays Society's homes in each Anglican diocese in England and Wales.

had accompanied many emigration parties on behalf of the Society for Promoting Christian Knowledge (SPCK), was commissioned to find a suitable property in Canada for use as a Receiving Home. By the end of 1884, a house at 117 Bowen Street, Sherbrooke, Quebec, had been acquired and named the Gibbs Home after its principal benefactor.

On 23 April 1885, the first party of girls to use the Sherbrooke home set sail from Liverpool accompanied by the Reverend Bridger and the home's future matron, Mrs H. W. Osgood.

Those selected for emigration had to be aged from 6 to 12, or else over 16 and trained in the Society's homes as domestic servants. They were to be in good health and of good character, and have the consent of their nearest relative. Although priority was given to girls from the Society's own homes, any vacancies could be offered to girls received from individuals, homes and institutions, and Boards of Guardians. They would travel from Liverpool to Quebec by the Allan Line of steamships.[7]

In 1887, following a donation of £500 from a Mr Richard Benyon, a second Receiving Home was set up in Sherbrooke, at 136 Bowen Street. The Benyon Home, as it was known, was used to accommodate boys.

In 1896, having reached the age of 67, Maria Rye decided it was time to retire and she handed over her homes in London and in Niagara-on-the-Lake to the Society. Thereafter, Niagara-on-the-Lake was used to receive girls, while the Gibbs Home, relocated to 21 Lawson Street, Sherbrooke, was used for the boys. The Benyon Home was then closed. From 1909 to 1911, the Society operated a Babies' Home in Winnipeg, Manitoba, which housed boys and girls aged from birth to 5 years.

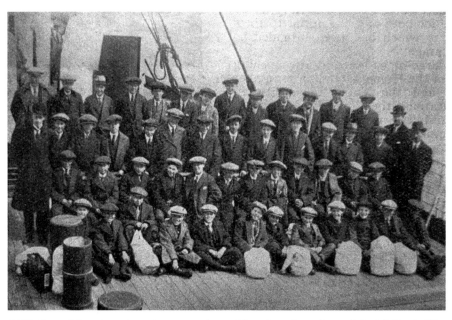

A Waifs and Strays emigration party bound for Canada on board the SS *Doric*. The group left Liverpool on 25 April 1924.

During the First World War, the Niagara home was taken over for military purposes and then disposed of by the Society in 1921. Three years later, a property was acquired at 661 Huron Street, Toronto, and named the Elizabeth Rye Home. It accommodated girls aged from 14 to 18 years who were trained for domestic service. The home closed in 1932.

The numbers of children migrated by the Society were always relatively modest. Between 1887 and 1914, the total numbered 2,250, with the largest contingent in any one year comprising the 90 girls and 65 boys who departed in 1907.[8] The First World War temporarily halted emigration but it gradually resumed afterwards. In 1928–30, 226 children left for Canada, with the overall total then having exceeded three thousand. The worldwide depression of the early 1930s brought emigration virtually to a standstill although a small number of boys from the Society immigrated to the Fairbridge home in Australia. The Gibbs Home in Sherbrooke was finally closed in 1933. A trickle of emigration continued, interrupted again by the Second World War, but its use was formally brought to an end in 1948.

Edward Rudolf's Departure

On 22 December 1907, Edward Rudolf finally fulfilled his long-standing ambition when he was ordained as a priest by the Bishop of London at St Paul's Cathedral. Thereafter, on visits to the Society's homes, he took considerable pleasure in being able to administer Holy Communion to the children and staff.

His mother died in 1910, a time which marked the beginning of a decline in his own health. However, he continued to work as hard as ever. Although he seriously considered becoming a parish priest, the demands it would have imposed on his time would have greatly reduced his involvement with the Society. He was, however, appointed as a Prebendary (a senior member of the clergy) at St Paul's Cathedral.

With increasing health problems, and rumblings in some quarters that he was 'past it', Rudolf took his retirement in September 1919, thirty-eight years since he had founded the Society. At a farewell celebration the following month at the Caxton Hall, the Bishop of London presented him with a cheque for £1,000 and a book inscribed with 3,000 names of those involved in the Society, ranging from the Archbishop of Canterbury to the children at the Society's smallest home.

Rudolf was succeeded as Secretary by the Reverend W. Fowell Swann, who held the post for five years. During Fowell Swann's tenure, the Society inaugurated what was to become an important aspect of its work – the provision of residential nurseries. This was in part a response to the rise in illegitimate births which had taken place during the latter years of the First World War – a trend that also subsequently resulted in the 1926 Adoption of Children Act. The Society's first nursery, the Edward Nicholl Home for Babies, was opened in Cardiff in 1918. The £21,000 cost of constructing the building was met by the Cornish MP, Sir Edward Nicholl, with the proviso that a similar amount had to be raised by the Society's supporters as an endowment fund for the running of the home. A second nursery, opened in Bristol in 1920, was named the Victoria Gibbs Memorial Home for Babies, commemorating a member of the same family that had helped fund the Gibbs Home in Canada. Others followed in Brislington and Plymouth.

After his retirement, Edward Rudolf made his home in Eastbourne but kept actively involved in the Society, remaining a member of all its committees. He also occupied himself in matters such as a detailed analysis of the expenditure on food in each of the Society's homes. He discovered, for example, that the annual cost per head at Knebworth was £22 4s. 8d., a figure that was disturbingly higher than that at any comparable home of £14 15s. 17d. All the time though, his health was declining. He also suffered the loss of his wife Emma in 1929, and his younger brother Robert in 1932. On 29 May 1933, he himself passed away.

The 1930s

The Society's Secretary since 1924, Dr A. J. Westcott, resigned in 1932, and his place was filled by the then Assistant Secretary, Mr W. R. Vaughan who had originally joined the Society as an office boy. In order to have a clergyman in the most senior ranks of the Society, a new post of Clerical Secretary was created in 1933 and its first incumbent was none other than Edward Rudolf's eldest son, the Reverend Cyril Rudolf, who was seconded for the purpose by the Community of the Resurrection to which he belonged.

Following Edward Rudolf's death in 1933, the Society launched the Rudolf Memorial Appeal to raise funds for new homes specializing in the care of children with behavioural problems or learning difficulties, what were then commonly referred to as 'backward' children. The first, a home for boys, was opened in 1935 in Clapham Park, followed in 1939 by one for girls in Dulwich.

Following the 1933 Children and Young Persons Act, the Home Office asked the Society to convert one of its homes into an Approved

School and the St Mary's Home for Girls in Felixstowe was selected for this purpose. After a further request, the St Augustine's Home for Boys in Sevenoaks was similarly redesignated.

In 1935, nine years after the passing of the 1926 Adoption Act, the Society made its first tentative steps into the field, with twenty-nine legal adoptions being arranged for children that had been in its care.[9] In the same year, the Society launched its Grants Scheme which provided financial support to help single mothers board out their children in their local area.

The Second World War

Other than a suspension of immigration to Canada, the First World War had relatively little impact on the Society. In the Second World War, things were rather different. Thirty of its then 106 homes were evacuated to safer locations, away from potential targets of enemy attack. With war having looked increasingly likely over the previous year, the plans for the evacuation were well prepared. For homes located in rural areas, the disruption was less severe, with sleeping quarters being moved to the ground floor as an example. Rationing severely restricted the supply of foods such as meat, eggs and cheese. To counter such shortages, homes often received parcels from America, Australia and Canada containing items such as jam, and dried milk and eggs.

One casualty of the German air raids was the Edward Nicholl Home for Babies in Cardiff which was hit by an incendiary bomb on 26 February 1941. Fortunately, the children and staff were safe inside the home's air-raid shelter. After several near misses, the Society's offices in Kennington were moved out to Eastcote in Middlesex, where they stayed for the rest of the war.

Not long after the start of the war, the Society realized that children under 5 presented a particular problem as they required much greater attention than older children and so were much more difficult to place as evacuees. Accordingly, a number of 'War Nurseries' began to be established, the first in February 1940 in Dallington, Northamptonshire. By the end of 1940, thirty War Nurseries had been set up, housing over a thousand babies and young children; two years later the number of War Nurseries had reached ninety-eight.[10]

The Post-War Years

As the war progressed, the Society began to consider what its direction and aims would be. Although it operated a large number of residential homes, fostering had always been viewed as the ideal form of care for children lacking their own family. In 1944, reflecting a shift between the balance of the two, the Hatton Home in Wellingborough became what was described as 'a reception and club centre for children boarded out in the vicinity. It is used for the rehabilitation of children before boarding out, and there is a percentage of "permanent boarders", children not suitable for foster parents. Provision is also made for visits by Old Boys'.[11]

The eventual aim of the scheme was to convert all suitable branch homes into Boarding-Out Centres, with a team of Boarding-Out Welfare Officers appointed to recruit and supervise the expanded number of foster homes. Other aspects of the Society's work were being put on a more professional footing with an increased emphasis on staff training and staff conferences. A staff training college was opened in 1947 in part of the Wellingborough home.

The planned change of emphasis was, however, hampered by the after-effects of the war. Homes which had been evacuated could not always simply just return to their old buildings. Some properties which had been requisitioned by the government were often slow to be handed back and were then discovered to have been damaged or neglected.

In 1946, the Society dropped the phrase 'Waifs and Strays' from its name and became the Church of England Children's Society. In the minds of the public, though, the old name was to linger for a great many years afterwards.

Also in 1946, in line with the general move towards housing boys and girls together, the Society opened its first mixed home in Bexhill.

The 1948 Children Act, resulting from the report of the Curtis Committee, decreed that adoption and fostering, rather than institutional care, should be given priority as the preferred outcome for children unable to grow up with their own families. The Act also gave considerable powers and responsibilities to local authorities, who were required to establish Children Committees and appoint Children Officers. In November 1949, A. R. Vaughan, the Society's Secretary since 1932, reached retirement age and – much to his chagrin – was forced to take his retirement. He could be consoled, however, by the thought that the changes introduced under his leadership, some pushed through in the face of considerable resentment, placed the Society in a good position to operate alongside the new council-run Children's Departments. After leaving the Society, he became General Secretary of the Fairbridge Society, an organization devoted to the emigration of children.

Into the Modern Era

Vaughan's successor as the Society's chief, a post which now became known as 'Director', was Colonel E. St J. Birnie. It was Birnie who was to oversee the transformation of the Society from a Victorian rescue mission to a modern agency which promoted the welfare of underprivileged children. Its aims and objects, revised in 1952, were closely modelled on the Curtis Committee's recommendations. Wherever possible, a child was to be enabled to remain with its mother or parents, with grants being provided to help cases of financial distress. If remaining with the parents or parent was inadvisable, and unless the help was of temporary nature, the next best option was adoption. The third best procedure was boarding out the child with foster parents, so that it could be brought up in a natural home. Where none of those was appropriate, children would be sent to one of the Society's homes, with every effort made to give them security. Any becoming available for adoption or boarding-out were provided with natural homes as soon as possible. The remainder stayed in the Society's homes until old enough to go out to work. The Society aimed to make its homes as non-institutional in nature as possible and to provide the children with as many outside contacts as possible, letting them gain self-reliance and knowledge of the outside world before leaving the Society's direct care.[12]

By the 1970s, great changes had taken place in social attitudes towards matters such as lone parenting and abortion. At the same time, there were fewer children entering children's homes or being placed for adoption by voluntary agencies because of increased activity by council social services departments in this area. As a result, the Children's Society made two major changes to the way it worked. The first, and most visible, was the closure of many of its children's homes. Second, it moved away from adoption and fostering and began to focus on helping young people solve their own problems.

A new initiative began in 1969 when the Society opened its first day-care centre at Foulkes House in South London. It offered support for one-parent families and those affected by illness, stress or severe poverty. The success of the venture led to the Society opening further centres across the country, often on the sites of its former residential nurseries.

The Society also opened a series of purpose-built family centres, often run in conjunction with local social services departments. In 1981, the Society's centenary year, twelve new family centres were opened in locations on large housing estates. Other projects at this period included the opening of toy libraries and soft play areas, and the setting up of information services to offer help with welfare rights.

In 1982, the Society shortened its name to just 'The Children's Society'. In 1986, the Society's headquarters moved from their long-standing home at the Old Town Hall in Kennington to its present-day base at Edward Rudolf House on Margery Street, London.

Today, the Children's Society continues to be one of Britain's leading child support agencies and currently runs over thirty-six children's centres in England, working in partnership with forty local authorities. It also has programmes up and down the country helping children and young people of all faiths who are struggling to cope.

Chapter 10

Occupational Homes

One of the first institutions providing care for the children of a particular occupation was Greenwich Royal Hospital School. It began life in 1712 as an extension of the activities of the Greenwich Royal Hospital, and provided for the maintenance and education of the orphans of mariners who had died in active service. However, it was not only obviously hazardous professions such as the military, the police force and railway workers that established orphanages. Homes were established for a wide range of other occupations such as teachers, actors and clerks.

Occupational homes were often founded by those who were themselves engaged in a particular business. Sometimes this might be as result of the death of a particular member, or as a development of an occupation's existing benevolent fund. The funding of a home was generally through the weekly contributions of members whose payments would then entitle them to benefit in the event of their own demise or permanent incapacity.

Clerical Homes

The Clergy Orphan Society was founded in 1749 to maintain and educate the poor, orphaned (i.e. fatherless) children of Anglican clergymen, with subscribers to its funds including George III. Initially placing children in existing establishments, the Society subsequently opened its own premises near Thirsk in Yorkshire, later moving to St John's Wood in London. In 1856, the boys were transferred to their own institution in Canterbury, with the girls moving in 1897 to Bushey, Hertfordshire. Both establishments still exist as modern-day independent schools.

The Home and School for Sons and Orphans of Missionaries, founded in 1842 in Blackheath, provided a home and education for the sons of missionaries connected with any British evangelical society. The Church Missionary Society established a home for the children of its members in 1850, its golden jubilee year, following a special appeal to finance commemorative projects. The Church Missionaries' Home, as it became known, was initially located in Islington but moved in 1886 to purpose-built premises in Limpsfield in Surrey.

Business Community Homes

In 1803, the business world entered the arena when the Friendly Society of Licensed Victuallers opened a school at Kennington Lane, Lambeth, for 'the maintenance and education of children of deceased or distressed licensed victuallers who have been subscribers during the time they were in business'. The property was rebuilt on a grand scale in 1836 and continued in use until the School moved to Slough in 1922, taking over the former premises of the British Orphan Asylum which had folded owing to financial difficulties.

Other establishments from within the business community included the Commercial Travellers' Schools in Wanstead (founded in 1845) and the Warehousemen and Clerks' Schools in New Cross (1854). Manchester's Warehousemen and Clerks quickly followed the lead of their London brethren and founded their own charity, initially placing children at an existing boarding school. Each of these groups went on to erect imposing purpose-built premises, the Commercial Travellers in Pinner, the Manchester Warehousemen in Cheadle Hulme and the London Warehousemen in Purley. In 1884, members of the drapery trade proposed the founding of a Drapers' Orphanage. However, a merger was eventually agreed with the Purley establishment which thereafter became Warehousemen, Clerks and Drapers' Schools.

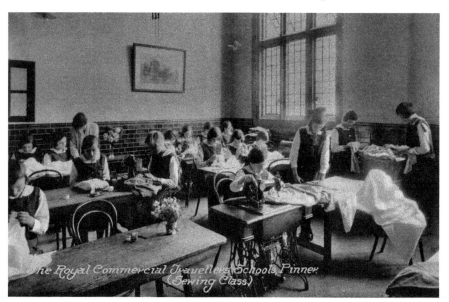

Girls at the Commercial Travellers' School, Pinner, cutting out material and sewing, early 1900s.

In 1903, the Furniture Trades' Provident and Benevolent Association founded its Orphan Homes in Radlett, Hertfordshire, and the Motor and Cycle Trades Benevolent Fund opened a children's home in Sydenham in 1921.

Sailors' and Soldiers' Homes

Reflecting Britain's considerable naval activities, the largest group of occupational institutions was that for the children of seafarers – this included not only sailors in the Royal or Merchant Navy but also those engaged in fishing and other maritime occupations.

The most ancient of these was the aforementioned Royal Hospital School in Greenwich, established in 1712, where up to 1,000 orphan boys were maintained, educated and prepared for naval service. Those eligible for admission were the sons of warrant officers, non-commissioned officers, petty officers and men of the Royal Navy, Royal Marines and the Royal Naval Volunteers who had been killed, drowned, or disabled in the service of the Crown. The sons of other seafaring persons, and men drowned on lifeboat service, could also be admitted. By Victorian times, applicants had to be between 11 and 14 at their time of admission, and were required to provide a certificate of the boy's birth, a certificate from a clergyman or schoolmaster as to his character and moral conduct, evidence of death of the parent, and an agreement signed by the boy and a parent or guardian that he would engage for service in Royal Navy or, if not physically fit to do so, would enter the Merchant Service and be enrolled in Royal Naval Reserve.

Other institutions for seafarers included London's Merchant Seamen's Orphan Asylum (1827), the Sailors' Orphan Girls' Home in Hampstead (1829), the Portsmouth Seamen and Marines' Orphan Schools (1834), the British Seamen's Orphan Boys' Home in Brixham (1859), the Liverpool Seamen's Orphan Institution (1868) and the Seamen's Orphanage for Boys in Southampton (1895). Hull was home to two nautical charities – the Sailors' Orphan Institution (1837) and the Hull Seamen's and General Orphanage (1866).

From around 1890, the Sailors' Orphan Society of Scotland operated several orphan homes in the Glasgow area, with a large purpose-built establishment being opened in Kilmacolm in 1899. The latter closed in the early 1930s when, it was claimed, the relatives of inmates, who had previously shown no interest in them, began to withdraw the children in order to receive a government allowance of 7s. 6d. a week for each of them.

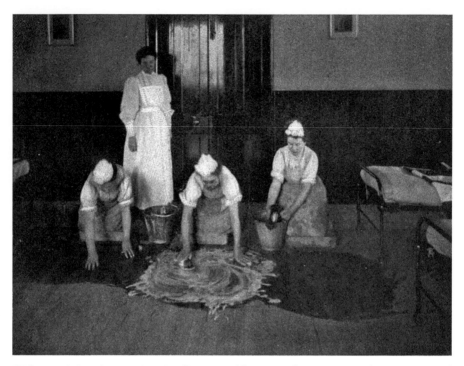

Girls receiving instruction in floor scrubbing at the Portsmouth Seamen and Marines' Orphan School, about 1908.

As well as homes for the orphans of naval personnel, a number were set up for other branches of the armed forces, in some cases coming in the wake of a major conflict. Institutions receiving the children of soldiers included the Soldiers' Daughters' Home in Hampstead (1855) and the Guards' Industrial Home in Westminster (1863). The Royal British Female Orphan Asylum in Devonport (1839) took the daughters both of soldiers and sailors, as did the Royal Victoria Patriotic Asylum for Girls in Wandsworth (1859), founded by Queen Victoria during the Crimean War. A Patriotic Asylum for Boys was also established but was closed in 1881. The admission policy at the London Orphan Asylum (1813) was that 'children whose parents have lost their lives in the army, navy, or marine and manufacturing services, are especially eligible'.[1] At the same institution, the children of domestic or agricultural servants, and of journeymen tradesmen, were all ineligible for admission.

Children with Scottish roots were served by the Caledonian Asylum, which was located in London rather than, as perhaps might be expected, north of the border. It was established in 1815, initially to provide support for Scottish children orphaned in the Napoleonic Wars which had ended that year. The charity subsequently broadened its remit to include 'the support and education of the children of soldiers, sailors, and marines, natives of Scotland, who have died or been disabled in the service of their country; and also the children of indigent and deserving Scotch parents resident in London'.[2]

The Soldiers' and Sailors' Families Association was founded in 1885 to assist the wives and families of servicemen. During the Second World War, SSAFA set up a number of homes to provide short-term accommodation for children of service families. The first was St Fillan's, in Heswall, opened after the heavy bombing of Liverpool in 1941. Another, Springbok House, in Great Baddow, near Chelmsford, was presented to SSAFA in 1949 by the people of South Africa in recognition of Britain's war efforts. Up to thirty children were accommodated, most staying only while their mothers were in hospital.

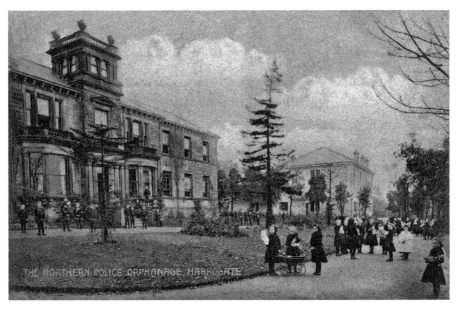

Children at play outside the Northern Police Orphanage, Harrogate.

Police Homes

Several institutions were founded to maintain and educate the children of police officers who had died in the course of their duties. The Metropolitan Police opened an orphanage in Twickenham in 1871. Its formally stated object was 'to afford relief to destitute orphans of members of the Metropolitan and City of London police forces; to provide them with clothing, maintenance, and education, to place them out in situations where the prospect of an honest livelihood shall be secured, and to grant compassionate allowances to those children, under 13 years of age, for whom there is no room in Orphanage'.[3] Growing problems in funding the home, coupled with an increase in the pensions provided to the widows and families of police officers, led to the Orphanage's closure in 1937.

Outside the capital, two national institutions were established. The Police Orphanage in Redhill, Surrey was opened in 1890, to serve the southern part of the country, with the St George's Police Orphanage in Harrogate, West Yorkshire, following in 1898 to provide for the northern counties.

Homes were also opened by two pairings of provincial forces. The Manchester and Salford Police Orphanage was established in 1889 but in around 1905 was absorbed into St George's in Harrogate. The Liverpool and Bootle Police Orphanage was founded in 1894 and, by March of that year, 1,400 out of the 1,700 officers in the two member forces had undertaken to contribute to its funds, paying a 5/- entrance fee to the scheme and a subscription of a penny each week. The Orphanage's premises in Woolton continued in operation until 1957.

Railway Workers' Homes

The children of railway workers were served by three homes. The first to be established, in 1874, was the Railway Servants' Orphanage in Derby – the location being chosen because of the town's central position and large railway works. Its initial premises were a small rented cottage where the first eleven children were received on New Year's Day 1875. Two years later, it moved into a large house with several acres of grounds on Ashbourne Road. The children attended local schools, the boys continuing to do so until they left the Orphanage. From the age of 13, however, the girls were kept at home and given training in domestic work. By the time they left, they were expected to know how to make their own dresses and other articles of clothing,

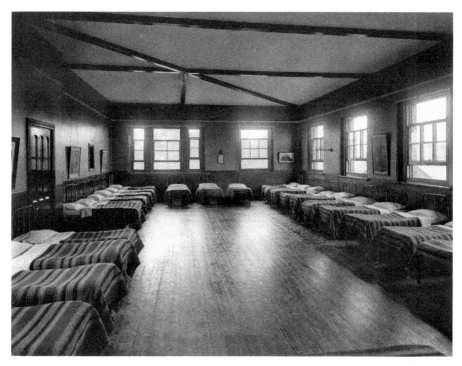

A dormitory at Derby Railway Servants' Orphanage. A basket for stowing clothes is placed under each bed.

to wash, iron and knit, and to cook a plain dinner. All the children received physical instruction in free movements, wand drill, club drill and exercises on the apparatus in the gymnasium. Both sexes were taught to swim. The boys were also taught either carpentry, shoe-mending or kitchen gardening, while the children kept small allotment gardens. Most of the boys went on to enter the railway service, while the girls became domestic servants, dressmakers, shop assistants or teachers.

In 1884, a shortage of places at the Derby home led to the creation of the London and South Western Railway Servants' Orphanage in Clapham – another railway hub. It was instigated by the Reverend Canon Allen Edwards, Vicar of All Saints, South Lambeth, who was also known as the 'Railwaymen's Parson'.

The third railway institution, the Webb Orphanage, was opened in 1912 in Crewe. It was intended for the children of employees of the London and North Western Railway (LNWR) who had accidentally died while working for the company. The Orphanage was funded out of a half-million-pound legacy from Francis William Webb. Webb had been an important figure in the LNWR, having risen from an apprentice in the locomotive works in Crewe to become the company's Chief Mechanical Engineer. Webb had also been keen to generate social improvement for the LNWR's workforce and for the town of Crewe, whose growth and economy was closely linked to the company's operation. The Orphanage joined other local amenities such as the town's Mechanics' Institute, Cottage Hospital, Queen's Park and Mill Street Hospice, which all owed much to Webb's efforts and financial help.

Teachers' Homes

In 1878, the National Union of Elementary Teachers established an Orphanage and Orphan Fund to 'erect, partially endow, and maintain an orphanage for the necessitous children of teachers, the term necessitous applying to a child whose father is permanently incapacitated'. In fact, two homes were subsequently set up. An orphanage for boys was opened in Peckham in 1884, later moving to Sydenham, where it became known as the Passmore Edwards Teachers' Orphanage in recognition of its main donor. A girls' orphanage was opened in Sheffield in 1887. After the boys' establishment was closed in 1951, the Sheffield establishment became mixed until its own demise in 1963.

Actors' Homes

The acting profession was served by two children's establishments, the Actors' Orphanage, opened in Croydon in 1906, and the Gracie Fields Orphanage, in Peacehaven, Sussex, opened in 1933. Though perhaps not an entirely typical institution, the Actors' Orphanage provides an interesting example of the evolution of a children's home.

In 1891, Mrs Kittie Carson, the wife of the editor of *The Stage* newspaper, founded the Theatrical Ladies' Guild to improve the welfare of women and children involved with the theatre. Initially, the Guild helped provide clothing to those in need such as young or unemployed actresses. In 1896, the Guild's growing concern with the welfare of children led it to establish the Actors' Orphanage Fund 'to board, clothe and educate destitute children of actors and actresses, and to fit them for useful positions in after life'.[4] The Fund's first President was the eminent actor, Sir Henry Irving.

As well as receiving donations and subscriptions from individuals, theatres around the country were invited to raise money by putting on a benefit matinée performance each year. Many actors and actresses also sold autographs for the benefit the Fund.

In 1906, the charity was able to establish its first orphanage in a leased property at 32–34 Morland Road, Croydon. Girls lived in one half of the semi-detached pair, and boys in the other. The children all attended local schools. The home was run by Mr and Mrs Ansell, but a growing catalogue of worries began to accumulate about the couple. At one inspection by the Visiting Sub-committee, concerns were raised about the lack of green vegetables being provided and also the poor state of the children's underclothes. In 1911, an outbreak of ringworm was discovered at the home. The poor quality of the food was again raised. It also appeared that two 15-year-old girls, Dolly Allport and Lilly Davis, were being allowed to wander the streets of Croydon unaccompanied. Most seriously, the mother of one of the girls at the home, a Mrs Beesley, was said to have raised complaints about Mr Ansell's conduct with her daughter. In December 1911, the Ansells were dismissed from their posts and the home temporarily closed, with the children being sent to stay with relatives or found alternative accommodation. The home re-opened in 1912 under the management of a new ladies' committee and with a new staff consisting of a matron, assistant matron, resident master, cook, two house generals, a between maid, a gardener and an odd job man.

With the lease on Morland Road due to expire in 1915, a search began for permanent premises. A suitable property was located in the shape of Langley Place, an old country house in Langley in Buckinghamshire, for the purchase of which the sum of £4,500 was raised. The orphanage transferred to its new home in the spring of 1915. There were again staffing problems with the home's master being dismissed owing to the boys' poor school reports, and the assistant master resigning over disagreements with the matron, whose own departure followed soon afterwards. Some stability was restored with the appointment of a new master, Mr Baumeister, who had overall control of the home, and the former assistant matron, Daisy Craft, being promoted to matron.

At Langley Place, the younger children were taught on the premises and the establishment became rather more like a charitably funded boarding school. The word 'Fund' was dropped from the charity's name which now became 'The Actors' Orphanage'. Fund-raising was still a major activity, however, with an important contribution coming from Penny Collections – a voluntary contribution of a penny in the pound of the income of working performers. An annual garden party at the Chelsea Royal Hospital also contributed to the finances.

In keeping with its theatrical roots, Langley Place had its own small theatre, known as The Bijou, with a stage, orchestra pit, scenery, lighting and dressing rooms. The home's Christmas pantomime was an annual highlight.

In 1934, Noël Coward became President of the charity and initiated many changes at the home. The buildings were redecorated, the grounds improved and a new boys' dormitory was built with the previous bunk beds replaced by single beds. He also ended the practice of cold baths and improved the food. When Coward visited the home, he came loaded with sweets and other treats and was often accompanied by well-known stars of stage and screen such as Mary Pickford, Rex Harrison, Edith Evans, Jack Hawkins, Sybil Thorndike and, in the 1950s, Marlene Dietrich.

In 1938, the orphanage moved again, this time to the Silverlands estate near Chertsey. With the onset of the Second World War the following year, the children – again thanks to the influence of Noël Coward – were evacuated to the United States where they remained until 1946.

In 1956, Sir Laurence Olivier took over as President with Richard Attenborough as his deputy. They instigated further changes at the home, working in conjunction with Mr and Mrs Slater who had taken charge of the establishment the previous year. The old dormitories were partitioned into individual cubicles each furnished with a new bed, small bureau and mirror. The children were divided into 'family groups', each containing a mixture of boys and girls of different ages and placed under the supervision of house parents. Each group had its own sitting room and dining room. The children were also allowed to choose some of their own clothes, listen to pop music and hold or attend Saturday night dances. Despite the changes, the tradition of Saturday morning chores continued – dusting and sorting laundry for the girls and shovelling coal for the boys.

In 1958, the cost of major repairs needed by the building, the declining numbers of children at the home, and the increasing difficulty of finding good staff at its isolated location resulted in a decision to close Silverlands. Instead, grants would be offered to the families of those children who could take them back, while others would be re-housed in two smaller properties in Watford. By 1961, a further dwindling in the number of children being supported by the charity led to the selling of the Watford houses.

In 1960, the Actors' Orphanage began moves to work in conjunction with Denville Hall, the actors' retirement home run by the Actors' Benevolent Fund. The two organizations merged to create The Actors' Charitable Trust (TACT) whose aim was to serve actors and their dependants.

In the early 1960s, a resurgence in demand for residential care led to TACT taking over the management of the Gracie Fields Orphanage in Peacehaven. As a rising singing star, Gracie had bought the property for her parents in 1928 but it proved too isolated for them. In 1933, Gracie donated the house to the Variety Ladies' Guild for use as a home for the children of deceased or impoverished actors. As well as paying the running costs of the home, which housed up to twenty-five children, Gracie remained a regular visitor, sometimes bringing along other show business folk for the children to meet. The Peacehaven home finally closed in 1967.

Chapter 11

Other Voluntary Homes

By 1930, the 'big three' organizations (Barnardo's, NCH and the Waif and Strays) were between them operating over 300 branches and housing more than 16,000 children. There were, however, a large number of other providers, many just running a single home, but with a few developing into organizations with a dozen or more establishments.

Mr Fegan's Homes

James William Condell Fegan was born in Southampton on 27 April 1852. His father, James, was employed at the Ordnance Survey headquarters in the city and was also a member of the Plymouth Brethren. Until the age of 10, young James was educated at home by his mother. In 1865, the family moved to London where he entered the City of London School. In 1869, he joined the office of a firm of colonial brokers, and the following year experienced an intense religious conversion while reading a Greek play. Sometime afterwards, while out distributing religious tracts, he encountered a group of boys from a nearby ragged school and subsequently began teaching at the establishment.

In September 1871, the strain of combining his job in the commercial world and long evenings teaching took its toll on his health and led to an enforced rest. While recuperating in Bognor, he came across a rough, ragged boy named Tom Hammond who made a strong impression on him. He brought Tom back to London with him and found the boy a place in an institution from where, eighteen months later, he immigrated to Canada. Fegan's ragged school pupils also opened his eyes to the dire conditions in which some of their acquaintances lived despite making a small income from working on the streets as shoe-blacks and match-sellers, or as mudlarks, grubbing along the river shore at low tide.

Fegan's response was to rent a nearby cottage for the sum of 5/- a week where some of the boys could come each evening and be taught whatever they could learn. Some were allowed to shelter there all night and continue their street occupations during the day. His thoughts then turned to the setting up of an Industrial Home which would provide training and work for the boys during the day as well as shelter at night. With a loan of £5 from each of four friends, the home was opened on 1 May 1872 at 112–114 High Street in Deptford. As the number of inmates grew, the home also took over 118 High Street. Further expansion came in 1879 when Fegan established the Little Wanderers' Home in Greenwich, followed in 1883 by a seaside branch in Ramsgate. At around the same date, he took a party of the boys for a summer camp in Downe, in Kent, where his now widowed mother was living. He was thus a pioneer of 'camping out', which was to become a well-established activity in boys' homes.

In July 1882, following the expiry of the lease on the Deptford property, Fegan moved his base to 95 Southwark Street, Southwark. Located on a broad thoroughfare running parallel to the Thames from London Bridge to Blackfriars Bridge on the Surrey side, Fegan later described the home as 'the most centrally situated of all Rescue Homes in the great city'.[1] The six-floor building could accommodate 150 boys who, rather than being sought out, came of their own accord or were brought by the police. The boys were taught various trades to enable them to earn their own livelihood. At one time, demand became so great that temporary premises had to be taken in an adjoining street for the shoemaking workshops. A printing department was also established in connection with the home.

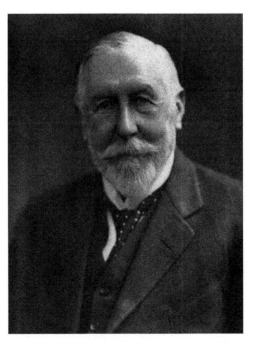

A portrait of camping-out pioneer James Fegan.

Like many child 'rescuers' of his day, Fegan saw immigration to countries such as Canada as a valuable way of giving his boys a better future. In the spring of 1884, he took his first party of ten boys to Canada and, having been greatly impressed by the opportunities he found there, went there again in the summer with a contingent of fifty whose expenses had been covered by a gift of £500 from Lord Blantyre who had become a valued friend and supporter. Fegan also received a donation from the MP Samuel Smith, director of the Liverpool Sheltering Home (see chapter 16). In Canada, Fegan was greatly assisted by William Gooderham, a wealthy distiller, who had himself originally come to Canada as part of an emigrant family. Gooderham initially provided Fegan's lads with accommodation in the Boys' Home he was building in Toronto, and 1886 funded a Distributing Home in the city, which Fegan shared with the Salvation Army.

In August 1889, Fegan married Miss Mary Pope, whom he had met nine months previously. After their marriage, the couple took up residence in two rooms at the Southwark Street Home, where they continued to live for the next twenty-three years.

In the 1890s, Fegan's glowing endorsement of a preparation called 'Homocea' regularly appeared in newspaper advertisements for the product. He vouched for having used the miracle medication on the boys at Southwark Street and had found it an effective treatment for all kinds of pain, accidents, inflammation, stiffness, sprains, mosquito bites, sore backs and broken heels. It had even helped his eyesight![2] It is not apparent whether Fegan received any remuneration from the manufacturers of 'Homocea' for use of his accolade.

By 1900, the location of the Little Wanderers' Home in Greenwich was increasingly felt to be unsuitable and it was relocated to some former school premises in Stony Stratford in Buckinghamshire.

In 1911, Fegan set up a training farm near Goudhurst, in Kent, to prepare boys for immigration to Canada. A cottage on the property was converted for use by Mr and Mrs Fegan.

As had been the case with the Greenwich home, the situation of the Southwark premises became increasingly undesirable and the location for a permanent replacement was found at 62–64 Horseferry Road, Westminster. The existing slum property on the site was demolished and a new building constructed. In it were housed the organization's General Offices, an Enquiry and Advisory Bureau, a Receiving Depot for new cases, and a Working Lads' Hostel.

In July 1920, in the wake of the First World War, Mrs Fegan announced that the charity would commemorate its approaching

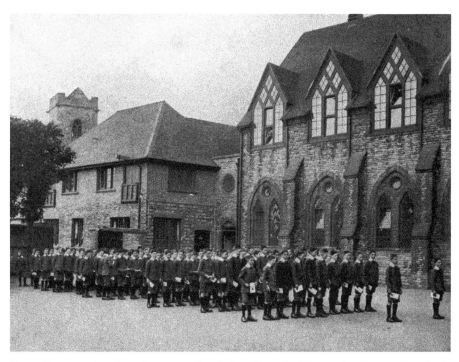

Boys line up in the playground of the Fegan's Home in Stony Stratford, Buckinghamshire.

Golden Jubilee by offering fifty new 'openings' – twenty for boys over 14 on the training farm in Goudhurst, and thirty for boys under 14 in the homes in Stony Stratford and Ramsgate. These would be for boys whose fathers had fallen in the war or become disabled through service in defence of their country, or 'whose widowed mothers – without any State allowance – are almost heartbroken in their hopeless struggle to provide bread, boots, etc., for their growing children in days of famine prices'.[3] Ten of the vacancies at Goudhurst would be aimed at redeeming 'Juvenile Bolshevists' who, it was hoped would be saved by a year's farm training, so that 'that they may become a strength and stay, and not a menace to the Commonwealth'.

James Fegan died at the Goudhurst farm on 9 December 1925. His widow, Mary, continued his work until her death at the farm cottage during a German air raid on 7 October 1943.

The present-day Fegan's charity continues its Christian-based work that aims 'to enable children, empower parents and equip churches'.

Quarrier's Homes

Scotland's largest children's institution was founded by William Quarrier, who was born in 1829 in Greenock in Renfrewshire. After his father, a ship's carpenter, died from cholera when William was just 3, the family moved to Glasgow. His mother took up laundry and sewing work to support William and his two sisters. At the age of 6, William began to contribute to the family income working a ten-hour day in a pin factory on Graeme Street for a weekly wage of one shilling. Two years later he became an apprentice to a shoe- and bootmaker, becoming qualified when he was 12 years old. When William was 17, he went to work as a shoemaker for a Mrs Hunter and began attending Blackfriars Baptist Church where he became a Christian. Six years later, he opened his own shoe shop, soon followed by two more. In 1856, he married Mrs Hunter's daughter, Isabella, and they had four children – Isabella, Agnes, Frank and Mary.

In November 1864, on his way home one evening, Quarrier was moved by an encounter with a young boy who had been selling matches, who was crying after his stock and night's earnings had been stolen by an older boy. He then took up the cause of street children, first by setting up a Shoeblack Brigade. The shoeblacks were provided with a shoe-cleaning kit and uniform, the cost of which they gradually

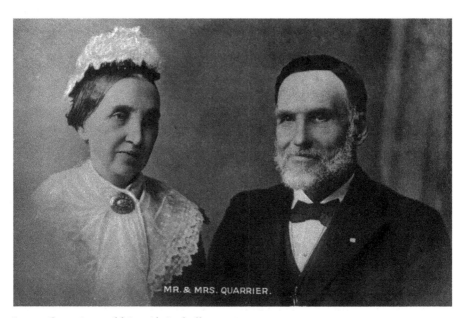

MR. & MRS. QUARRIER.

James Quarrier and his wife Isabella.

repaid from their earnings. They were also required to attend school classes in the evening and a Sunday School. A similar scheme followed for another group of Glasgow children who sold newspapers on the city's streets. A third enterprise, the Parcel Brigade, provide a team of uniformed parcel carriers who charged their customers a rate of 2d. per half mile, or 3d. a mile. The three brigades had a joint headquarters – the 'Industrial Brigade Home' – in Glasgow's Trongate. The schemes were not as successful as Quarrier had hoped and were wound up within a few years.

During his work with the brigades, Quarrier met Annie Macpherson, an advocate of sending poor children to start new lives Canada, who convinced him of the benefits of such work. In 1871, Quarrier had raised sufficient funds to open a home for orphaned children at 10 Renfrew Lane, Glasgow, and by the spring of the following year, thirty-five children were ready to immigrate to Canada. As the numbers of children grew, a second house was rented on Renfield Street where the girls were housed, while the boys were moved to a mansion in Govan named Cessnock House. The girls later moved to the Newstead and Elm Park homes in Govan. A night refuge and mission hall were also set up in Dovehill, replaced in 1875 by a new building in James Morrison Street, which became known as the City Orphan Home.

Quarrier's ultimate vision was to take poor children completely away from the city streets. Instead of the traditional large monolithic institutions, he was influenced by the new cottage homes developments that were beginning to receive interest during the 1870s, where groups of children were housed in a 'village' of family-style homes.

In 1876, with money raised from a growing band of supporters, Quarrier bought the 40-acre Nittingshill Farm located between Bridge of Weir and Kilmacolm. Building work commenced with the £1,500 cost of each children's house being met by further donations from friends. The site, known as the Orphan Homes of Scotland, opened in 1878 and eventually included around fifty houses together with everything needed for it to be a self-contained community including a school, church, infirmary, post-office, general store and even its own fire station.

As well as his work with children, Quarrier contributed to his country's healthcare provision. In 1896, he set up Scotland's first sanatorium for tuberculosis patients on a site adjacent to the Homes. This was followed by the creation of the 'Colony of Mercy' providing care for sufferers of epilepsy. However, the latter was not to open its doors until after William Quarrier's death which took place in October 1903.

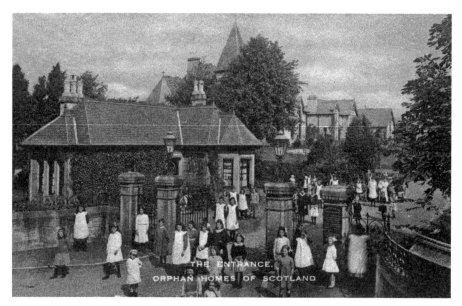

Children at the entrance to the Orphan Homes of Scotland, early 1900s.

During the 1920s and 1930s, the Homes housed up to more than 1,500 children at any one time. The establishment continued operating much as Quarrier had begun it until the early 1980s, with over 30,000 children being cared for during that period. Of that total, over 7,000 had immigrated to Canada or Australia. However, with changes in child care practice and legislation, numbers residing at the village declined steadily from the 1970s onwards. The Quarriers organization now directs its efforts to providing a wide range of social care services throughout Scotland.

The Manchester and Salford Refuges

The charity known as the Manchester and Salford Boys' and Girls' Refuges (MSBGR) was founded 1870 by Leonard Kilbee Shaw and Richard Bramwell Taylor who were Sunday School teachers at St Ann's Church, Manchester. It aimed to help the city's homeless and destitute children without any requirement for payment or recommendation.

Shaw and Taylor raised money from local businesses and opened their first home for boys at 16 Quay Street, Deansgate. Boys up to 16 years of age were given a bed for the night and found work as office messengers and bootblacks. In 1871, the home moved to what became known as the No. 1 Central Home on 14 Francis (or Frances) Street, Strangeways. The premises, formed from four three-storey houses and an adjoining yard, were gradually extended and by 1883 could accommodate up to 120 boys. The location was also the charity's headquarters until 1920 when the site was sold for £16,000.

The MSBGR's No. 2 Home was opened in 1874 at 214 Lower Broughton Road, Manchester, and housed seventeen working boys, aged 14 to 18. The No. 3 Home, at St John's Place, 107 Great Clowes Street, Lower Broughton, Manchester, was opened in 1876 with similar accommodation to the No. 2 Home. 1876 also saw the opening of the No. 4 Home at 8 Camp Street, Lower Broughton, Manchester. It housed up to seventeen homeless boys, aged 14 to 18, mainly those engaged as 'hookers' in cloth warehouses.

The work schemes supported by the MSBGR steadily grew to include the City Messenger Brigade, Boy Commissionaires, Newspaper and Shoeblack Brigades, and the Caxton Brigade of Boy Colporteurs. The Caxton Brigade sold cheap and 'pure' literature on the streets, with members paying a small subscription for use of a uniform and of the Refuge's reading-room and lavatory. Some of the boys in the charity's care were placed on the training ship *Indefatigable*.

In around 1875, a Home for Little Boys – those below the age of 10 – was established at 34–36 Great Ducie Street. In July 1877, the home moved to new premises at Johnson Street, Cheetham. The property, formerly two adjacent private houses, had a communal playground but was otherwise run as two separate family-style groups, each with sixteen boys under the care of a matron. The boys attended the St John's School and St Luke's Sunday School.

An Open-All-Night Shelter was established in 1878 at 14 Major Street, Manchester. It provided temporary accommodation for up to twenty children, aged from 5 to 15, who had been found without proper guardians or suffering under cruel treatment. By the later 1890s, the Shelter was located at 1 Chatham Street, off Piccadilly.

On 26 October 1881, Mr Henry Lee, MP, opened the charity's Boys' Rest, Lodging House and Coffee Room in Angel Meadow. The premises were the former Old Victory Coffee House at the junction of Angel Street and St Michael's Place.

In 1878, an 'Industrial Branch' for twenty-eight girls aged 9 to 16 was opened at 'Heathfield' on Broughton Lane, Manchester. It closed in 1894.

On 11 November 1882, the Bishop of Manchester formally opened new accommodation at 4–12 George Street, off Cheetham Hill – what was then described as 'a very healthy and pleasant district'. The first four houses, all for boys, were respectively named the 'Garnett',

'Crossley', 'Higgins' and 'Atkinson' homes after benefactors whose gifts had enabled their purchase. The fifth home, for girls, was funded by money raised by the girls of Lancashire and Cheshire and named the 'School Girls' Home'. A sixth house, 2 George Street, joined the others after its existing tenancy had expired and was named 'Langworthy'. The houses, which could each accommodate sixteen children, all had playgrounds at the rear and small lawns at the front, planted with shrubs. The whole block was purchased and fitted up at a cost of about £5,000. Children admitted to the homes were required to be under 10 years of age and with both parents dead. Each of the homes was in the charge of a matron who was known to the children as 'mother'.

An emigration home for girls, known as Rosen Hallas, was opened in 1886 at the corner of George Street and Cheetham Hill. It gave the girls training in domestic skills prior to their being migrated to Canada. An adjacent cottage was used as a convalescent home. A boys' emigration home was established in 1891 on Great Ducie Street. The Boys' Refuge also took over the work of the Gordon Boys' Home – a home for delinquent boys on Chester Road, Cornbrook, which had got into difficulties owing to financial mismanagement.

In 1883, the charity established its first premises outside Manchester, with the opening of a seaside convalescent home in Lytham, which in 1915 moved to Old Colwyn in north Wales. The charity's Home for Crippled and Incurable Children was opened in 1890 at a property known as Bethesda on Coke Street, Cheetham Hill.

In around 1891, a block of properties at 68–80 Great Ducie Street was taken over by the charity, just around the corner from the Central Refuge for Boys on Francis Street. The block housed the Boys' Refuge Depot (i.e. stores for the Refuge), the Boy's Emigration Home, a Brigade Boys' Home (for boys working in the Shoeblack and Messenger Brigades) and a new Working Boys' Home to replace the old homes in Lower Broughton.

Another new home was opened in 1896 at Tetlow Grove House, Cheetham Hill, to house up to twenty motherless children, aged from 5 to 15 years. Motherless children were a group for whom relatively little provision existed. Many of the children at the home were subsequently able to return to their fathers, perhaps following a remarriage. By 1904, the service had been transferred to the Higgins Home on George Street.

In 1920, the MSBGR began to create the Children's Garden Village on the Belmont House estate in Cheadle, where the facilities included a sanatorium and recreation hall.

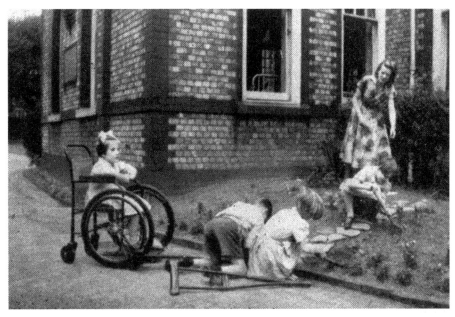

Children gardening at the Manchester and Salford Refuges' Bethesda Home, 1940s.

After the Second War, the general trend towards smaller, community-based, family-group homes led the charity eventually to establish four of these, namely Linden, 64 Station Road, Cheadle Hulme (1958), Lerryn, 66 Parsonage Road, Heaton Moor, Stockport (1960), Highlea, 1 Crossacres Road, Gatley, Stockport (1963) and Lockhart House, 51 Parsonage Road, Didsbury. These were partly funded by the sale of property from Manchester's Jubilee School, a struggling charity which the MSBGR took over in 1958. In the same year, the Bethesda Home moved out from Leicester Road to make use of the growing amount of vacant space at the Belmont site.

In 1960, the organization changed its name to the Boys' and Girls' Welfare Society and in 1966 merged with the Invalid Children's Aid Association through which it inherited the Taxal Edge Convalescent Home on Macclesfield Road, Whaley Bridge. Belmont House was disposed of in 1983 owing to financial difficulties.

Renamed the Together Trust in 2005, the charity now offers care, support and special education to children, adults and families, including those with particular physical, behavioural or learning difficulties.

Miss Sharman's Homes

Charlotte Sharman was born in 1832 in Southwark and was brought up in a deeply religious Evangelical atmosphere. After visiting a workhouse to see some orphans whose parents she had known, she took a growing interest in the plight of such children, especially girls, many of whom ended up living on the streets. For some that she encountered, she found homes with the families of friends, or paid for their care with foster parents. Others she passed on to the homes run by George Müller in Bristol. After writing a pamphlet about the need for a home to care for such girls, the encouragement and financial support that she was offered led her to set one up herself.

The home was opened in May 1867 in a rented house next door to her mother's residence in West Square, Southwark. The first residents were ten small girls under the care of a teacher who acted both as a matron and governess. A year later, the children numbered forty-two, necessitating a move to a larger house. In May 1869, there were eighty children and a second property was taken on. By 1870, four houses in and around West Square were occupied. In 1871, the homes included a nursery branch with thirty-six children at 32 West Square, one for another thirty-six children aged from 5 to 8 at 23 West Square, an infirmary at 44 West Square, and a large house known as The Mansion at 14 South Street (now Austral Street) with ninety-three residents. The Mansion, provided at a modest rent by the Vicar of Botolph, was also used as a school.

When the poor state of The Mansion led to an order for its demolition, Sharman decided to erect her own building on the site and in 1875, the foundations stone of what was to become the 'Orphans' Nest' was laid by the Duchess of Sutherland. The north wing of the new home was ready for use in the following May although it took until 1884 for the whole building to be completed.

Any applicant for admission was required to be an orphan and destitute and, if over 12 years of age, to provide a satisfactory reference as to her character. All cases were strictly investigated and, except in extreme cases, they were admitted in rotation. Admission was free, except for cases supported by special subscriptions. Inmates were 'carefully instructed in superior needlework, and receive[d] a plain English education' to equip them for domestic service.[4] The institution was described as 'Protestant inter-denominational', with the girls attending chapel on Sunday mornings and church in the afternoon.

As well as the Orphans' Nest, a small home was maintained in operation at 21 West Square. In 1891, Miss Sharman was living next door at 20 West Square with her companion, Louise Colley, and her adopted daughter Charlotte, then aged sixteen. She also established branch homes in Gravesend, Tunbridge Wells, Newton Abbot and Hastings. An 'Educational Branch' was located in St Michael's Road, Stockwell.

Miss Sharman died in December 1929, at the age of 97. She worked up until the end, typing her letters herself. It was said that during her life she had cared for more than 2,700 children and had received more than £320,000 in charitable donations to support her work.

The Austral Street building is now occupied by the Imperial War Museum's photographic archive.

Spurgeon's Orphan Homes

Born in 1834, Charles Haddon Spurgeon became a charismatic preacher and leading member of a denomination known as the Strict Baptists. In 1867, inspired by the work of George Müller in Bristol, he established an Orphan Home for Boys in Stockwell, in south-west London. The scheme of the Orphanage, in Spurgeon's words, 'proposed to do away with all voting and canvassing, with the wasteful expenditure necessitated thereby, and also to form the orphans into large families instead of massing them together on the workhouse system'.[5] The latter idea proved helpful in the raising of funds, with many donors each giving a sum sufficient to build one house, while the smaller gifts of less wealthy sympathizers provided the means to build the dining-hall and other common rooms. As a silver-wedding gift from her husband, a Mrs Tyson gave £500 to build a house which was named 'Silver-wedding House'. A merchant provided £600 for a 'Merchant's House', and Mr William Higgs and his workmen promised to build a 'Workmen's House', while Mr Thomas Olney and his sons agreed to provide 'Unity House' in memory of Mrs Unity Olney. The Baptist Church donated £1,200 as a testimonial to Spurgeon for the erection of two 'Testimonial Houses'; a 'Sunday School House' was given by the Tabernacle Sunday School, and a 'Student's House' by the ministers trained at the Pastors' College which Spurgeon had founded in 1857.

Each house or villa at the orphanage was run along the lines of a family home, with a Christian 'mother' or matron at its head. Family prayers were conducted each morning before the duties of the day began. For the sake of economy, however, meals were taken in the institution's communal dining-hall. It was a deliberate policy that the

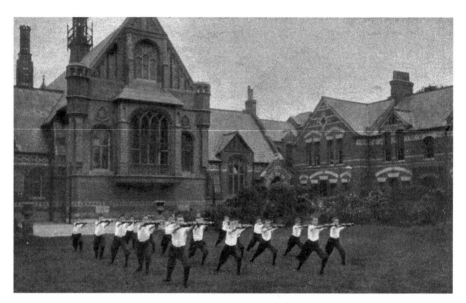

Boys perform a drill with dumb-bells at Spurgeon's Orphanage, Stockwell.

inmates of the home should not wear a distinctive uniform that would identify them as charity children. Instead, they wore ordinary clothing, all slightly different from one another.

The boys were given a 'good English education' which aimed to fit then for positions in the world of commerce, although manual skills such as carpentry also featured in the curriculum. In religious matters, the home was Christian but non-sectarian and the denominations represented among the children included Church of England, Baptist, Congregational, Wesleyan, Presbyterian, Brethren, Roman Catholic, Moravian, Bible Christian, Society of Friends and Salvation Army.

A girls' section was added to the orphanage in 1879, and a large house with grounds was acquired at 193 Clapham Road adjoining the Orphanage. By 1882, the entire institution covered more than four acres and housed 250 boys and 250 girls. The girls' homes were run along similar lines to the boys', the most notable difference being that the girls dined in their various houses rather than in a communal hall. The girls, as was usually the case in such homes, received training in domestic skills.

Children were required to be between the ages of 4 and 11 at the time of their entry to the home. 'Unhealthy, deformed, imbecile and illegitimate' children were ineligible for admission and inmates were dismissed if a surviving parent remarried.[6]

The home's band of choirboys and hand-bell ringers regularly gave performances over a large area and the collections among the congregations made a useful addition to the institution's income.

In 1939, at the onset of the Second World War, the children were moved to St David's, a large house and grounds in Reigate. A further move came in 1951 when the Homes transferred to purpose-built premises in Birchington, Kent, where the children's houses were arranged in a distinctive zigzag layout. The Birchington home was closed in around 1979.

The charity founded by Charles Spurgeon, now known simply as Spurgeons, continues to provide a wide variety of support for disadvantaged young people and their families. It also runs a number of visitor centres at prisons for anyone visiting a prisoner, including those with children.

The Orphanage's former Reigate premises are now used by the Surrey Fire and Rescue Service, while the Birchington houses have now been adapted for private residential use.

The Blackburn Orphanage

James Dixon was born in Annan, Scotland, in 1855 but his family subsequently moved to Blackburn, Lancashire where he worked as a journeyman joiner. In 1881, after witnessing boys sleeping out all night on cellar steps, he and a friend founded the town's Bent Street Ragged School, contributing a pound a week from his own wages to support the establishment.

In April 1884, following repeated requests from boys at the school to be allowed to sleep on the forms, a Boys' Home was opened in rented premises on Feilden Street. The following November, a Girls' Refuge was added on Barley Lane.

In 1886, Dixon began raising funds for the building of an orphanage for the town, contributing £50 of his own savings. A site was found on the Whalley Road, near Wilpshire, to the north of Blackburn and, in August 1889, the foundation stone was laid by the Mayor of Blackburn. The formal opening, in May 1891, was performed by Miss Derbyshire, of Limefield, Blackburn, who had donated the cost of the land. The building initially housed thirty boys and fifteen girls, aged from 4 to 12 years. A second block was added in 1904 which was then used as the girls' accommodation.

No charge was made for those entering the Orphanage. The most needy and deserving cases were chosen by the ten-strong committee elected annually from those subscribing two guineas or more. Priority was given to children who had lost both their father and mother.

Dixon continued to superintend the Orphanage until his death in 1936. The surviving girls' block is still occupied by the charity Dixon founded, now known as Child Action Northwest, which continues to support local children and young people in need.

Homes for Motherless Children

The Homes for Motherless Children organization was set up in 1896 by the evangelist Robert Thomson Smith. Smith had a particular interest in helping children who had lost their mother through death or other circumstances but had a father who was able to provide for their care.

The first children's home to be opened by Smith was at 13 Hogarth Place, Old Chiswick. A friend of the Mission, Mr J. R. Wooster, offered to pay the rent of the house for a year. One of the rooms was furnished by another friend, Mr Donaldson, in memory of his mother, and Mrs Donaldson performed the opening ceremony on 5 March 1896. The first child to be admitted was Alice Castledine, followed by a small disabled boy named Brown. The home was soon full, with fifteen children in residence. Those placing a child in the home were required to make a weekly payment of four shillings. Smith subsequently opened further homes in Ealing, Hanwell and Hounslow.

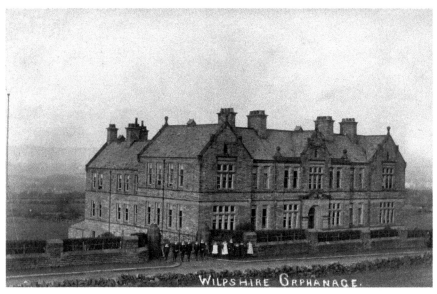

Children stand outside the Blackburn and District Orphanage in Wilpshire, near Blackburn.

Mrs Smyly's Homes

Ellen Franks was born in Dublin in about 1815. In her late teens she became involved in visiting sick poor children in hospital or in their homes. She was married in 1834 to Josiah Smyly, a surgeon at Dublin's Meath Hospital, with whom she had twelve children. When her own family demands had begun to recede, she returned to her charitable endeavours and in 1852 set up a daytime Ragged School in a stable loft on Townsend Street, Dublin. Here, up to 200 children were provided with breakfast (bread and cocoa) and dinner and given a basic education together with Bible lessons and hymn singing.

Ellen Smyly's work soon progressed to establishing residential children's homes, beginning with the Ragged Boys' Home (1852), Coombe Ragged Day School and Boys' Home (1853), Girls' Home and Infants' Day School (1854), The Bird's Nest (1859), Elliott Home for Waifs and Strays (1872) and Home for Big Lads (1883). Her activities influenced other child care workers, notably Thomas Barnardo, who became a close friend.

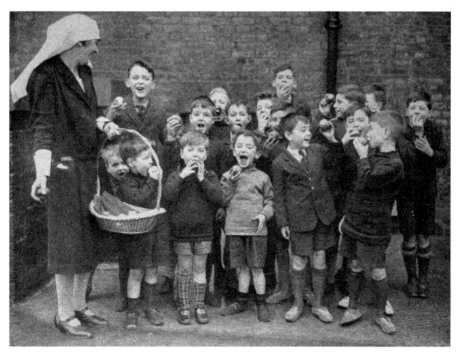

Boys at a Home for Motherless Children enjoy a gift of apples sent from Canada by a former resident.

In the early 1900s, the Smyly organization moved to what became its long-standing base at 21–22 Grattan Street, Dublin. After Smyly's death on 16 May 1901, her work was continued by her daughters Ellen, Annie, and Harriet. Like many similar organizations, Smyly's migrated some of its older children to Canada, eventually establishing its own reception and distribution home, The Coombe, in Hespeler, Ontario, in 1905.

Children's Aid Society

The Children's Aid Society (CAS) came into being as a division of the Reformatory and Refuge Union (RRU), a body formed by managers of reformatory institutions in 1856. The RRU's membership gradually grew to include the managers of other institutions such as Industrial Schools, Certified Schools and Magdalen Homes, and its activities included the holding of conferences and issuing of useful publications. The RRU also provided financial assistance to member institutions through its Metropolitan Refuge Fund, later renamed the Children's Aid and Refuge Fund. This operation subsequently became known as the Children's Aid Society, a title that was sometimes used as an alternative name for the whole Union.

The CAS gradually expanded its activities and by 1906 employed seven officers 'seeking out and saving, day by day, little children from destitution, degradation, and neglect'. The children it rescued were then placed in children's institutions across the country.[7] The Society also migrated children to Canada and by 1890 had its own receiving home in Winnipeg.

It was only in the 1920s that the CAS began to run a small number of its own residential homes in England, with around a dozen eventually being established or taken over from other operators. All were located in London and the Home Counties and included the Blunham Babies' Home in Bedfordshire and the Knotley Hall Approved School in Chiddingstone Causeway in Kent.

The CAS ceased operation in around 1966 and was absorbed by the Barnardo's organization.

The Caldecott Community

The Caldecott Community was founded in 1911 by Miss Leila Rendell. It began life in St Pancras, London, as a day nursery for children whose families, through poverty or neglect, could not care for them. It subsequently became the Caldecott Community, moving several times before settling in 1947 in Mersham-le-Hatch, near Ashford, Kent. Now renamed the Caldecott Foundation, it provides residential care and other facilities for young people aged 5 to 18 years.

Gifts and Endowments by Individuals

Like the previously mentioned Webb Orphanage for the children of railway workers, a number of other homes were funded by gifts or legacies from wealthy individuals:

- The Female Orphan Asylum in Brighton was established in 1822 by the Chevalier François de Rosaz 'to clothe, board, and instruct gratuitously, poor orphan girls who have lost both parents'. When de Rosaz died in 1876, he left money for the founding of a Protestant Orphan Asylum in the town. In 1893, after many years of legal wrangling, the de Rosaz legacy reverted to his earlier establishment, whose formal name then became the Female Orphan Asylum and De Rosaz Protestant Orphan Asylum.
- The Royal Orphanage in Wolverhampton was founded in 1850 by local lock manufacturer John Lees to provide a home for children left orphaned by a serious outbreak of cholera in the town. The subsequent development of the institution was, however, largely funded by public donations.
- The Crossley Orphan Home in Halifax, West Yorkshire was founded in 1857 by Francis, John and Joseph Crossley – three brothers from a local carpet-manufacturing family. In 1887, following a £50,000 endowment by Manchester yarn merchant, Thomas Porter, the establishment was renamed the Crossley and Porter Orphan Home and Schools.
- Mason's Orphanage in Birmingham, financed by local industrialist Sir Josiah Mason, opened in 1858 in purpose-built premises in Erdington. It admitted only legitimate boys and girls who had lost both parents. Such was the demand for places that, two years later, on a new site, Mason laid the foundation stone for a much larger building to house 300 children. When the new building opened in 1868, the original premises were converted to almshouses for the elderly.
- Crowley's Orphanage for Poor Girls, also in Birmingham, was founded in 1869 following a £10,000 gift and a further £1,000 legacy for the purpose made by Thomas Crowley, a timber merchant. Its object was 'to maintain and educate poor orphan

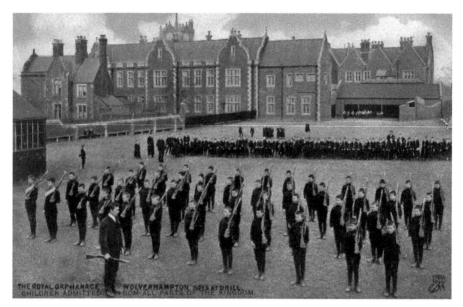

Boys at drill at the Royal Orphanage, Wolverhampton, early 1900s.

girls who were born in wedlock, and who have lost both parents, and afterwards to place them in situations'.

- Chadwick's Orphanage, in Bolton, Lancashire, was opened in 1874 to house up to eighty girls. It resulted from a gift of £22,000 by Dr Samuel Taylor Chadwick of Southport who for many years had practised in Bolton.

- Eden's Orphanage, also in Bolton, was funded by James Eden, senior partner in the bleaching firm Eden and Thwaites. At his death in 1874, Eden left £10,000 for the building of a home for destitute infant children, both of whose parents were dead. A further £40,000 was left to be invested, with the income used for the maintenance of the orphanage, the support and clothing of the children, and the payment and support of the staff.

- The Aberlour Orphanage in Morayshire began life in 1875 after Miss Macpherson Grant promised to fund construction of the home, complete with its own school, church and rectory, if Canon Charles Jupp – a man with a particular interest in the care of orphaned and abandoned children – agreed to become her personal chaplain. Following Miss Macpherson's death in 1877, its continued development owed much to an £8,000 legacy by Mr William Grant of Wester Elchies.

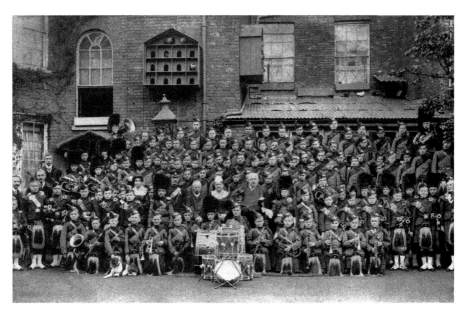

Inmates in their Highland regalia at the Gordon Boys' Orphanage, Dover. The home's founder, Thomas Blackman, stands at the centre.

- The Harris Orphanage in Preston, Lancashire, resulted from a legacy by Edmund Robert Harris, a wealthy lawyer from the town who died in 1877. Having no heirs, he bequeathed the then massive sum of £300,000 to set up a trust for philanthropic purposes in memory of the Harris family. A third of the money was used to found the orphanage which was built as a cottage homes development.
- The Pendlebury Orphanage in Stockport, Cheshire was established in 1882 following a £100,000 legacy by Sir Ralph Pendlebury, a former Mayor of Stockport and mill owner. After Pendlebury died in 1861, it took twenty years for his legatees to settle on the Orphanage scheme.
- The Nutter Orphanage for Boys, in Bradford, West Yorkshire, was established in 1884 following a £10,000 legacy from Joseph Nutter, a Halifax man who had been successful in business in Bradford. Nutter stipulated, however, that the money would be given only if the site and building were provided by the efforts of others within twelve months of his death – a condition that was successfully met.

- The Gordon Boys' Orphanage and Home in Dover was founded in 1885 by local philanthropist Thomas Blackman. It was one of several establishments to be named after General Charles George Gordon who had died in the siege of Khartoum earlier that year. The home was noted for its drum and fife band which, adopting the Gordon tartan, performed in full Scottish regalia. Blackman remained as director of the Orphanage until his death in 1921.

Chapter 12

Religious Homes

A large number of children's homes were run by religious groups and organizations, usually as part of a wider range of social care activities. The Church of England's involvement was primarily through the Waifs and Strays Society, with several Anglican sisterhoods also involved in working with 'penitent' single mothers. The Methodists made a major contribution via the National Children's Home, while the Jewish and Quaker faiths also operated a small number of establishments. It was the Roman Catholic community, though, that perhaps made the most vigorous contribution to this sector.

One of the main driving factors behind this involvement was the belief that only a Catholic institution could be relied upon to nurture and protect a Catholic child's faith. State-run institutions, such as the workhouse, were officially Anglican, and might expose a child to anti-Catholic hostility or prejudice, while many children's charities were avowedly Protestant and had a proselytizing mission.

Roman Catholic Homes

Although there were a number of Catholic children's homes operating in Ireland from at least the eighteenth century, the same was not the case in England where the Catholic faith was the subject of much persecution or discrimination in the centuries following the Reformation. One of the first to be established was the Catholic Female Orphanage in Liverpool, a city with a large Catholic population. The Orphanage began life in 1816 as a privately run house at 96 Mount Pleasant, moving in 1845 to Falkner Street where its operation was taken over by an Irish order of nuns, the Sisters of Mercy. Elsewhere in the country, in towns such as Birmingham, Manchester, Nottingham, Carlisle and London, education for destitute Catholic children was provided in charitably funded schools. By the 1830s, St Patrick's Charity School, in London's Soho district, also operated an orphanage.

Government funding for elementary schools began in 1839 but it was a requirement of receiving a grant that establishments had to agree to use a Protestant Bible. This effectively barred Catholic schools from benefiting from the system until this restriction was relaxed in 1847.

Catholic provision for orphan and other deprived children considerably benefited from the arrival in England of a number of religious orders such as the Sisters of Mercy in 1839, the Sisters of the Good Shepherd in 1841, the Daughters of Charity of St Vincent de Paul in 1847, the Sisters of Nazareth in 1851 and the De La Salle Brothers in 1855. Another group, the Irish Christian Brothers, had opened a school in Preston in 1825, followed by around another twenty over the following two decades. However, the Brothers were opposed to state funding and the inspections that went with it and eventually withdrew from England.

While many convents set up small orphanages in part of their premises, some orders founded separate and often quite large institutions, such as the Nazareth Houses operated by the Sisters of Nazareth. In other instances, sisterhoods offered, or were invited, to run establishments set up by other bodies.

A significant impetus for the setting-up of homes for Catholic children was provided by the 1862 Certified Schools Act which allowed Poor Law authorities to board out children in establishments run by voluntary bodies. A number of existing Catholic homes became licensed for this purpose, and many new ones were subsequently established.

The Daughters of Charity of St Vincent de Paul

The Daughters of Charity were founded in 1633 by a French priest, Vincent de Paul, and a widow, Louise de Marillac. They undertook a variety of work among the poor of Paris, running hospitals, working in prisons, and establishing homes for orphaned children. The Order quickly grew and by the time of de Paul's death in 1660, had more than forty branches across France.

The Order's first venture in England was in Salford in 1847, where they visited the sick and held classes for factory girls. However, in a wave of anti-Catholic agitation, the sisters were physically attacked and their house set on fire. In 1849 the sisters retreated to Paris but returned to England in 1857, to Sheffield, where they again began visiting the sick and running evening classes for girls. A member of the Sheffield community went on to take charge of the St Joseph's Reformatory for Girls, opened in Howard Hill, near Sheffield, in 1861.

In 1859, the Order founded a large establishment in Westminster. In 1863, it moved into a newly building on Carlisle Place, known as St Vincent's, which included an orphanage, workroom and day middle school for girls, a crèche, a night school for men and boys, and a soup kitchen. A second crèche, for the children of milk-women, was opened on Beaumont Street, Marylebone, in 1868. Another London orphanage, the St Vincent's School for Boys, was established in 1887 at Mill Hill.

St Elizabeth's School in Bullingham, near Hereford, was opened in 1861 and as well as an orphanage for poor girls included a 'middle-class' girls' school. In 1875, a second establishment, St Vincent's, was opened in Hereford itself for children between the ages of 3 and eight. In 1870, back in the Sheffield area, the sisters took on the running of the St John's Institution for the Deaf and Dumb. Their association with the establishment continued after it moved to Boston Spa in 1875, only finally ending in 1998.

The Order's presence in Scotland began in 1864 with the opening of the Smyllum Orphanage, Lanark. It catered for Catholic children aged from 1 to 14 years at their time of admission. In 1888, 440 children were in residence. Like its English counterparts, the Orphanage was supported by the parochial boards that administered Scotland's poor relief system. By 1890, forty-two boards had placed their Catholic children at the institution. The Orphanage inmates included blind and deaf-mute children. In 1890, it was noted that deaf-mutes at the establishment were 'taught by the new system of articulation and lip reading by a teacher specially taught in London to teach the dumb'.[1]

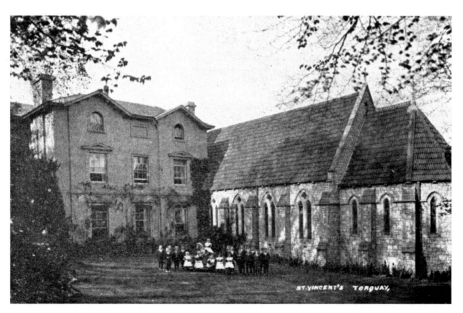

Children in the garden of St Vincent's Orphanage, Torquay, one of the homes run by the Daughters of Charity.

St Elizabeth's School for Girls was opened in Salisbury in 1868, becoming the Order's first Industrial School in 1875. Another girls' Industrial School, St Joseph's, was opened in 1892 in Darlington. It was followed in 1894 by one for boys in Elswick, near Newcastle upon Tyne. In 1896, the sisters were asked to run the new Bishop O'Reilly Memorial School for Catholic Boys in Preston.

In the twentieth century, the Order ran several dozen other establishments for children and young people in England and Scotland. These included the St Joseph's Hospital for the Mentally Handicapped in Rosewell (opened 1924), St Vincent's Open-air School in Dover (1927), Our Lady's Hostel for Business Girls in Willesden (1928), the Mother and Baby Home in Salford (1932) and the St John's Home for Girls in Erdington, Birmingham, which became an Approved School in 1948.

In line with other providers, the Order saw a steady decline in demand for places at its homes and by the end of the 1980s had closed virtually all its children's establishments in Britain.

The Daughters of Charity should not be confused with the Society of St Vincent de Paul, a lay organization founded in Paris in 1833 and established in England in 1844. Its object was 'to visit the poor, and to assist personally at their homes by moral and material help as far as possible'. The English branch was particularly involved in children's provision in the Catholic Diocese of Westminster. The Society is still very active today.

The Sisters of Nazareth

In 1851, following a request from the Archbishop of Westminster, Cardinal Wiseman, to the Little Sisters of the Poor in the French town of Rennes, where they ran a house to care for the elderly poor, a party of four nuns was sent to set up a similar establishment in London. Among the group was Victoire Larmenier, who was appointed the group's Superior. After several changes of premises, the sisters raised the necessary funds for the buildings of their first permanent establishment, opened in 1857 in Hammersmith. As well as the elderly poor, the home provided accommodation for destitute and orphan Roman Catholic children.

In 1861, the group separated from the Little Sisters of the Poor and formed a new order known as the Sisters of Nazareth (or sometimes the Poor Sisters of Nazareth). Larmenier, who then adopted the name Mother St Basil, is now regarded of as the founder of the Order. By the time of her death in June 1878, Larmenier had founded a further eight Nazareth Houses in the British Isles, although one of these was retained by the Little Sisters of the Poor.[2] Among these early establishments were those in Cardiff (1872), Southend (1873), Pontypridd (1874), Oxford (1875), Nottingham (1876) and Belfast (1876). As at Hammersmith, most of the Houses provided accommodation both for necessitous children and for the elderly poor.

Larmenier's successor was Margaret Owen (Mother Mary of the Nativity), under whose leadership the Order expanded across the world. When she died in 1908, an additional twenty-two Nazareth Houses had been founded, their locations including Australia, New Zealand and South Africa, as well as Britain. The head of the Order from 1909 to 1922 was Henrietta Greene (Mother Clare of the Cross), during whose tenure eleven more Houses were established.

Although a few of the homes, such as Cardiff, were for girls only, the more usual practice was for both boys and girls to be admitted from around the age of two. The girls remained until they were 14 or so, many then going into domestic service. On reaching the age of 7, the boys were usually transferred to other Catholic-run homes, with a small number of Nazareth Houses, such as Southend and Swansea, also accommodating older boys. At Belfast, a separate building housing up to 300 boys was opened in 1899.

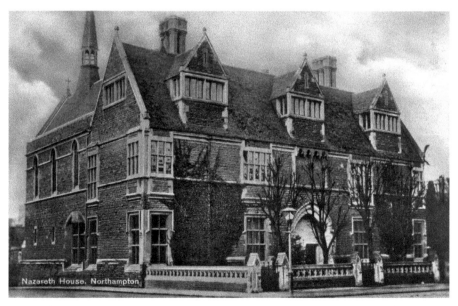

The Nazareth House established in 1875 on Barrack Road, Northampton. It housed up to 60 girls.

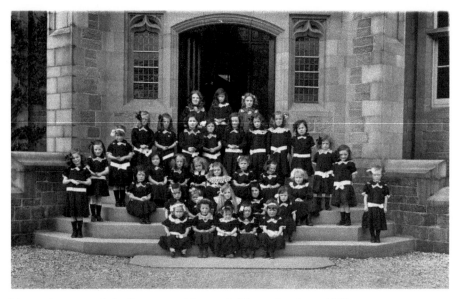

Young inmates of the Lancaster Nazareth House in about 1913.

Life for Nazareth House inmates followed a typically regimented routine. The usual day for the girls at the Newcastle home began with the ringing of the rising bell, washing and dressing. After Mass and Communion came breakfast in the refectory, with trays of plates being distributed by those on 'server' duty. The girls then returned to their dormitories, changed into their work clothes, formed into groups with a senior in charge of each, and proceeded to the various areas of the building to do cleaning and polishing. After work, they put on their school clothes and went down to the classrooms. Apart from a lunch break, lessons continued until 3.45 p.m. when 'collation' – a tea of bread and jam – was served in the refectory. A period of games and play ensued, outdoors whenever possible, briefly interrupted by the ring of a bell for the saying of the Angelus prayer. After attending Benediction in the church, dinner was followed by a recreation period which ended with a bell for the saying of the rosary. It was then back to the dormitories for night prayers and bed.[3]

The Order's Superior General from 1946 to 1958 was Honora Hough (Mother Emmanuel Mary) who introduced a broader range of professional training for the sisters including nursing, child care, catering and teaching. During this period, the Order also participated in a child emigration scheme and set up a reception and training home in Geraldton in Western Australia.

The end of the Order's provision of residential child care, at least as far as the UK, Ireland and Australia were concerned, came during the tenure of Ursula Patricia Comerton (Mother Mary Austin) which ran from 1976 to 1988. The steadily growing use of fostering had led to a fall in the demand for residential places, something which affected all the traditional children's home operators. The Nazareth Houses' long tradition of providing care for the elderly continued, however, an area which continues to expand. Nonetheless, more recent years have seen the closure of a number of the UK Nazareth Houses including those in Kilmarnock, Aberdeen, Middlesbrough, Nottingham, Ditton, Wrexham, Bexhill and Isleworth.

Sisters of Mercy

The organization that became the Sisters of Mercy was founded in Dublin in 1827 by Catherine McAuley, an Irish Catholic laywoman. With the help of a large inheritance, she erected a 'House of Mercy' on Baggot Street, Dublin, which provided shelter and education for poor women and girls. On the advice of the Archbishop of Dublin, she established a religious order to develop the work, with herself and two colleagues becoming the first Sisters of Mercy in 1831. In 1839,

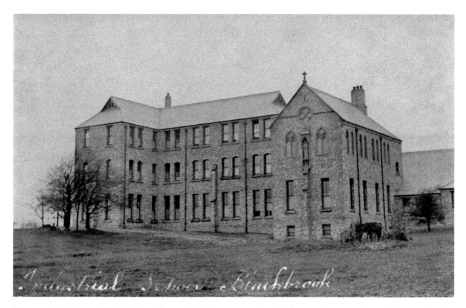

From 1869 to 1876, Blackbrook House in St Helens, Lancashire, housed the Liverpool Catholic Girls' Reformatory, run by the Sisters of Mercy. It later became an Industrial School in the charge of the Sisters of the Sacred Heart of Mary, then an Approved School run by the Daughters of Charity.

the Order opened its first convent in England, in Bermondsey, South London. Others followed in Handsworth, near Birmingham, in 1841 and in Mount Vernon, Liverpool, in 1843.

The care of children always featured prominently in the sisters' activities. As previously noted, they took over the running of Liverpool's Catholic Female Orphanage in 1845. In 1851, they established the Maryvale Orphanage in Perry Barr, Birmingham. The Order operated a number of Certified Schools including the Orphanage for Girls, Wigton, Cumberland (1882), St Joseph's, Aston, Birmingham (1884), St Mary's, West Croydon, Surrey (1886), St Mary's, Eltham, Kent (1887), St Mary's, Westbury on Trym, Bristol (1897) and St Anne's, Orpington, Kent (1903). They also ran several Reformatory, Industrial and Approved Schools including Blackbrook House, St Helens, Lancashire (1869), St Mary's, Eltham, Kent (1871–86), St Vincent's, Whitstable, Kent (1899) and St Joseph's (later renamed St Teresa's), Bristol (1916).

Catholic Conflict with Barnardo

Thomas Barnardo had a very proprietorial attitude to those who came into his care, believing that having rescued a child from destitution or neglect, he was not going to hand it over at the whim of the child's parents of relatives. Accordingly, anyone who placed a child with his organization was required to sign a written agreement handing over the complete care of the child, for an unspecified number of years, during which it was to be brought up in the Protestant faith. For any child who might be a candidate for immigration to Canada, there was an additional form giving permission for him or her to be sent overseas. Legally, however, these forms carried no weight if a parent or nearest relative decided to demand the return of a child. Unsurprisingly, perhaps, given his Irish Protestant background, Barnardo's reluctance to hand over children was particularly vigorous when it came to his dealings with the Roman Catholic community.

In 1887, following a number of disputes and legal proceedings, Barnardo came to an agreement with the Archbishop of Westminster, Cardinal Manning, that any Catholic child applying for admission to one of his institutions would first be referred to the Cardinal or one of his agents to deal with. Where Barnardo refused to compromise, though, was with children whom he had already received into one of his homes.

Barnardo's failure to return Catholic children in his care, even to a demand from a parent, resulted in legal proceedings against him which, in two cases, he fought – unsuccessfully – as far as the House of Lords. However, the publicity given to the proceedings provoked a major debate about the rights of a mother to retain her child even if she could be demonstrated to be totally unfit as a parent. The power to take legal custody of a child in certain situations had been given to boards of guardians (the local Poor Law authorities) in the 1889 Poor Law Act, for example where the child had been deserted or where a parent had committed an imprisonable offence against it. Owing much to Barnardo's vociferous campaigning, the 1891 Custody of Children Act made further inroads into the inalienable rights of a parent over its child. The Act provided that where a parent had abandoned or deserted their child, or allowed it to be brought up by another person at that person's expense, or by a board of guardians, then the return of the child to its parent could be refused.

The 1891 Act provided Barnardo with some consolation for his unsuccessful (and expensive) legal wranglings, and also resulted in an uneasy truce with the Catholic authorities. Antagonism between Barnardo and some quarters of the Catholic community was slow to wane, however. The opening of his Ever Open Door in Edinburgh was viewed with antipathy in Roman Catholic quarters of the city, and the London-based *Catholic Herald* published a story alleging cruelty and neglect by James and Janet Graham, the managers of the home. Although the Grahams successfully sued the paper's publisher, Charles Diamond MP, Barnardo decided to withdraw from Edinburgh and the home was closed shortly afterwards.

Catholic Diocesan Organizations

England's Catholic diocesan hierarchy had been restored in 1850 by Pope Pius IX and Catholic social care work was largely organized and co-ordinated at a diocesan rather than national level. Most Catholic dioceses eventually formed 'rescue' societies to promote the care of destitute or orphaned Catholic children and young people. Prominent among these were the Liverpool Catholic Children's Protection Society (founded in 1881), the Salford Catholic Children's Rescue Society (1886), Southwark's Catholic Rescue Society (1887), the Birmingham Diocesan Rescue Society (1902), Westminster's Crusade of Rescue (1899), the Clifton Catholic Rescue Society (1904) and the Leeds Diocesan Rescue and Protection Society (1910). In most cases, these Societies grew out of activities that had been taking place for many years previously. For example, the Westminster Crusade of Rescue could trace its origins

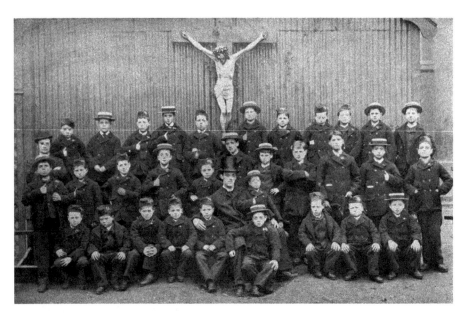

St Vincent's Home for Catholic Boys on Harrow Road, Paddington. The home's manager, Father (Lord Archibald) Douglas, is seated centre.

back to the founding in 1859 of the St Vincent's Home for Destitute Boys in Brook Green, Hammersmith. In many cases, dioceses also supplemented their own facilities by means of sharing arrangements with neighbouring dioceses.

Many of these societies are still in operation although having undergone a number of name changes over the years; for example, the Leeds Diocesan Rescue and Protection Society was renamed the Catholic Child Welfare Society in 1982, the Catholic Social Welfare Society in 1985 and Catholic Care in 1993. More recently, following the failure of these groups to obtain exemption from providing adoption services to same-sex couples, they have been forced either to sever their formal links with the Catholic Church, to accept no new adoption clients, or to close down altogether.

The early development of these organizations often owed much to the work of particularly energetic and committed individuals such as Father James Nugent in Liverpool, who set up shelters, residential homes and training schools for street children, also becoming a pioneer of children's emigration. The leading figure in the Birmingham Diocese was Father George Hudson, in whose memory the Diocesan Rescue Society was renamed the Father Hudson's Society in 1984.

Father Hudson's Homes

Father George Vincent Hudson was born in 1873 in the parish of Bredon in Worcestershire and was ordained as a Roman Catholic priest in 1898. He then became parish priest at Coleshill, near Birmingham, where he remained for the next thirty-six years.

A Catholic children's home already existed in Coleshill when Father Hudson arrived. St Paul's, located on the High Street, had been set up by the Birmingham Diocese in 1884. As a Certified School, it took Catholic boys from the children's cottage homes at Marston Green operated by the Birmingham Poor Law authority. The establishment also provided a day school for Catholic boys living in the area.

At Coleshill, Father Hudson became closely involved in working with deprived and destitute children. This led to his appointment, in 1902, as Secretary and Administrator of the newly formed Birmingham Diocesan Rescue Society ('for the Protection of Homeless and Friendless Catholic Children' to give its full name). The Society was soon dealing with hundreds of cases a year, with the children involved ending up in a variety of destinations. Some went to existing Catholic children's homes, including the St Vincent's Working Boys' Home in Birmingham. Others were placed in Poor Law schools, some were passed to other rescue societies, and some were migrated to Canada.

Right from the start, the Society had intended to open its own boys' home since the existing homes in the diocese provided fewer places for boys than for girls. The plan took a major step forward in April 1904 when Father Hudson was able to take possession of a two-acre site on Coventry Road, Coleshill, opposite St John's Church. The new building, known as the St Edward's Home, was opened on 6 November 1906, with Father Hudson appointed as its administrator and Mother Aloysia Marie Fleming as Mother Superior.

In common with many other children's agencies of the time, the Rescue Society saw emigration as an important option for providing a better future for the children that came its way. On 15 October 1903, Father Hudson took a party of eleven children to Canada – the first of thirty such trips he was to make. Following the formation of the Catholic Emigration Association (CAE) in 1904, Father Hudson became treasurer and then secretary of the organization, with the emigration of all Catholic children from England and Wales being administered from Coleshill. Children arriving in Canada initially stayed at the St George's reception home on Richmond Road, Ottawa, established in 1896 by the Southwark Catholic Emigration Association. Boys were

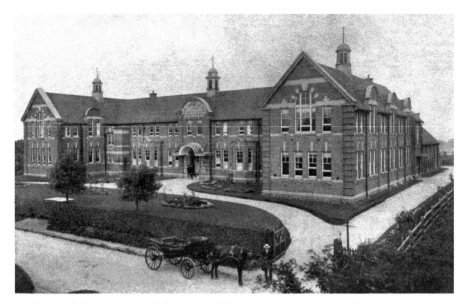

St Edward's Home, part of the Father Hudson's site at Coleshill.

placed mainly on farms while the girls generally went into domestic service. Catholic immigration to Canada came to a halt in 1932, by which time around 11,000 children had been sent by the CAE.[4]

In 1908, increasing concern about the health of the children at Coleshill, especially tubercular conditions, led to the opening of a temporary infirmary, known as St John's. A permanent establishment, St Gerard's Hospital, was opened at the site in May 1913. It could accommodate thirty-seven children and was open to children from all the Catholic children's homes in the Birmingham diocese and also Catholic children from workhouse infirmaries. To deal with the large proportion of tubercular cases, an open-air ward was soon added. During the First World War, St Gerard's became a Voluntary Aid Detachment (VAD) hospital, with soldiers being accommodated in the main building and children in the open-air ward. After the war, St Gerard's developed as a tuberculosis sanatorium and also provided orthopaedic care. The facilities were expanded with the addition of an operating theatre, additional open-air ward, X-ray department and chapel building. In around 1930, a nurses' home, known as St Mary's, was erected between St Edward's and the school building.

Up until 1914, the boys from St Edward's attended the school that operated at the St Paul's Home. In October of that year, the St Edward's Elementary School was opened at the main Coventry Road site.

The school was taken over by the local Education Board in 1925, from which date it admitted local children as well as those from the home.

In 1910, an extension known as Our Lady's Home for Babies was added to St Edward's to house children between 3 and 5 years in age. In 1923, two cottage homes, named St George's and St James', were erected at the south of the school building, with accommodation for a total of a hundred boys aged from 5 to eleven. The boys were expected to help with the household chores, with the older ones helping to dress the younger ones in the morning.

In 1931, a new educational facility, St Philomena's School of Social, Domestic and Commercial Science, was opened in conjunction with St Gerard's Hospital. The following year, two sisters who had trained at Guy's Hospital, London, opened a school of massage in the premises of the former St Paul's Home.

The first accommodation for girls appeared in 1931 with the opening of St Joan's Home. From the age of 11, the girls attended what was now the Catholic Central School at the St Paul's School site. They could also participate in the St Philomena's School training courses which included the study of household management, cookery, needlework, dressmaking, the care of linen and clothing, laundry work, first aid, home nursing and hygiene.

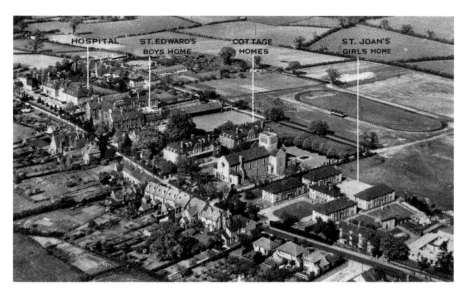

A 1930s bird's-eye view of the Father Hudson's site indicating the different sections of the buildings.

Father Hudson died in 1936 and was buried near the St Edward's Home.

After the war, there was a brief renewal of interest in migration, this time to Australia. By the time all emigration from Catholic homes ceased in 1956, a total of 133 children from Father Hudson's Homes had gone to Australia.

When the time came for boys to leave one of the Coleshill homes, those who had found work in Birmingham were generally housed in the Rescue Society's St Vincent's Working Boys' Home on Moseley Road, Bordesley. In 1945, for those more inclined towards agricultural work, the Society bought Priory Farm in Studley, Worcestershire. Its 250 acres were farmed by ten boys who learned the skills of cereal growing, dairying, poultry keeping, and market gardening. The Priory farmhouse provided them with hostel-style accommodation under the supervision of a resident warden. In 1948, the Manresa hostel on Vernon Road, Edgbaston, was opened to provide accommodation for girls leaving the Society's care and entering the employment market.

In the 1970s and 1980s, a growing emphasis on fostering, adoption and family support led to a fall in demand for residential places and a gradual closure of the homes. St Paul's School closed in 1970, with the newer buildings being demolished. The original St Paul's Home was converted for use as a mother and baby home but closed in 1985 and the property sold. The cottage homes closed in 1980 although, during the winter of 1981/2, they provided a temporary home for forty Vietnamese refugees. St Edward's closed in December 1981, with the remaining boys being transferred to the St Andrew's Home. In 1986, the St Michael's and St Catherine's wings of St Joan's were adapted to house sixteen young people with physical and learning difficulties. However, St Joan's was finally closed in 1989 and the buildings demolished in around 1997. St Gerard's Hospital closed the following year.

Father Hudson's Care, as the Society was renamed in 2015, is now a broadly based social care agency and still has its headquarters at Coleshill.

Anglican Orders

The Church of England's main provider of residential children's care was the Waifs and Strays Society, whose homes were run by lay staff. There were, however, a number of other Anglican establishments for children and young women, many of these operated by Anglican orders of nuns. The most prominent of these groups were the Community of St Mary the Virgin (founded 1848, and based in Wantage, Berkshire), the Sisterhood of St John the Baptist (1852, Clewer, Berkshire), the Sisters of St Margaret (1855, East Grinstead) and the Sisters of the Church (1870, Kilburn, London). By the 1930s, the establishments run by the Sisters of the Church – also known as the Church Extension Association – included 'Orphanages of Mercy' for orphans and friendless children in Kilburn, Liverpool, Eastcombe, Clevedon, Brondesbury and Broadstairs. They also ran children's convalescent homes in Broadstairs and Lytham St Annes.

Some orders, such as the Community of St Peter the Apostle, in Horbury, near Wakefield, ran Penitentiaries or Magdalen Homes for repentant 'fallen' girls and young women, usually in conjunction with the Church Penitentiary Association. Many also established training homes and refuges for those considered to be in moral danger. More information on these institutions can be found in chapter 19.

The Salvation Army

In 1865, William Booth founded an Evangelical Christian movement in the East End of London. Originally known as the Christian Revival Association, it was renamed in 1870 to become the East London Christian Mission, subsequently shortened to the Christian Mission. The group was reorganized and renamed in 1878 to become the Salvation Army – affectionately known as the 'Sally Ann'. The Army, with 'General' Booth at its head, adopted a military-style uniform and 'Articles of War' which included renouncing the use of alcohol. The Army also eschewed religious sacraments such as baptism and communion, considering them unnecessary.

In addition to its religious crusading, the Army gradually became involved a variety of social welfare activities. One of the earliest, in May 1884, was a women's refuge at 212 Hanbury Street, Whitechapel, opened as part of a campaign to rescue young women from prostitution. The Army's first night shelter was opened in 1888 at West India Dock Road in Limehouse, with many others soon following. The shelters provided a warm place to sit for the night upon payment of a penny, and so became known as 'penny sit-ups'. In 1889, a night shelter for women was opened at 194 Hanbury Street, originally at a charge of 2d. a night, later raised to 3d. after the London County Council made the provision of sheets compulsory.

In 1895, The Nest, a home for sexually abused girls, was established at 10 Springfield, Upper Clapton. In the same year, a shelter for boys was opened at 31 Fetter Lane, and at around the same date the Army took over Sturge House on Bow Road, a former Barnardo children's home. The home accommodated boys aged 14 to 18 who stayed at the home for a while, were taught and fed, and then helped to find work.

In around 1895, Ivy House, at 271 Mare Street, Hackney, was opened as a twenty-five-bed maternity hospital for unmarried mothers, most of whom were between 15 and 20 years old. The hospital catered for women both from London and elsewhere.

As well as providing immediate medical care, the Army found work in service for many young women so that they could support their child. Where possible, they were placed in households where only one servant was kept, so that they would be spared embarrassment from the others finding out their 'secret'. The Army also made efforts to locate the children's fathers, with the aim of obtaining financial support, either voluntarily or through a bastardy order.

At the end of the First World War, to help the plight of widows and their children, the Army arranged for a total of 1,769 women and 1,019 children to emigrate to new lives in Canada, Africa, Australia and New Zealand. In the late 1920s, the Army arranged the passage of several consignments of emigrants to Australia on the SS *Vedic*. By

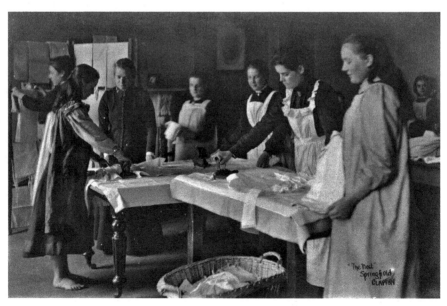

The Nest – the Salvation Army's home for sexually abused girls in Clapton, East London. An officer supervises inmates ironing.

1938, the overall total of men, women and children settled overseas by the Army's Emigration Department was almost 250,000.[5]

The Church Army

The Church Army was founded in 1882 by the Reverend Wilson Carlile as an evangelistic mission for the Church of England, working in the slum areas of London and other cities. The Church Army's Social Department aimed to 'raise the hopeless outcasts of society' by providing labour, rescue and lodging homes, of which around 120 were eventually established in London and the provinces, together with a farm colony in Hempstead in Essex. Although relatively little of the Church Army's work was with children, it operated a number of Magdalen and preventive homes for young women (see chapter 19).

Jewish Homes

One of the earliest establishments for Jewish children was the home founded in 1703 by the Spanish and Portuguese Jews' Orphan Society. Its object was the 'maintaining, clothing, housing, educating, and apprenticing of orphan children of the Spanish and Portuguese Jews';[6] in fact, admission appears to have been limited to boys. The institution occupied a series of premises in the London area, finally settling in Maida Vale in around 1900.

The Jews' Hospital (or 'Neve Zedek') was founded in the East End of London in 1795 following a proposal by Abraham and Benjamin Goldsmid, members of a prominent Jewish banking family. As with other 'hospitals' of the period, the institution was not intended as a medical facility but rather a refuge for poor and needy members of the Jewish community in the area, its object later described as being for 'the support of the aged, and the maintenance, education, and employment of youth'.[7] The brothers soon raised sufficient funds to open the establishment although problems with officialdom delayed its inauguration for a number of years. A property was eventually purchased on the north side of Mile End Road, Whitechapel, and formally opened at the end of June 1807. It initially accommodated five old men, five old women, ten boys and eight girls.

By the late 1850s, however, the decaying state of the premises led to plans being made and funds raised for a new building. An eight-acre site on the west side of Knights Hill Road, Lower Norwood, was given for the purpose by Mr and Mrs Barnet Meyers. The foundation stone of the new hospital was laid by Sir Anthony de Rothschild in June 1861, and the building was consecrated in February 1863, by the Chief Rabbi, the Reverend Dr Adler. The Jacobean-style building could accommodate 220 children.

In 1868, the establishment was accredited for operation as a Certified School, allowing it to receive workhouse children placed by boards of guardians. Children boarded out by Guardians were charged at a fixed weekly rate – in 1890, this was 6/- per week. Admission could also be gained via a twice-yearly election of the charity's governors and subscribers. Annual subscribers of 10s. 6d. had one vote at each election, while donors of £10. 10s. were given two votes. Children seeking admission had to be of Jewish parentage, with boys aged from 9 to 11 years of age and girls from 8 to twelve. Orphans were admitted from the age of two. Children received a 'plain education' and were either apprenticed to a trade or found suitable situations. By 1900, the establishment could accommodate 350 children.

In 1876, the Hospital merged with the Jews' Orphan Asylum (see below) and became known as the Jews' Hospital and Orphan Asylum.

In 1928, the institution was renamed the Jewish Orphanage, then in 1956 the institution became known as the Norwood Home for Jewish Children. In line with the general trend to family-group accommodation, Samuel House and Stephany House were erected in the orphanage grounds and seven further houses acquired in the area, including 17–19 Chatsworth Way, West Norwood. The main building was finally closed in 1961 and demolished two years later.

The Jews' Orphan Asylum began life in 1830 in London's East End after a poor couple named Assenheim died in the cholera epidemic of that year. A cucumber seller named Abraham Green raised money in the Jewish quarter for the support of their three small children, with his brother-in-law, Isaac Valentine, going on to establish a permanent institution. The Asylum's first premises, opened in 1831, were at Leman Street, Whitechapel. In 1846, it moved to purpose-built accommodation at St Mark's Street, Goodman's Fields, Whitechapel. In November of the same year, the new building was fortunate to escape serious damage when the nearby Garrick Theatre was destroyed by fire. In 1869, the Asylum was accredited as a Certified School. After its merger with the Jews' Hospital in Norwood in 1876, the St Mark's Street premises were closed.

Other Jewish institutions included an Industrial School for boys at Uxbridge Road, Hayes (opened in 1900), one for girls at Stamford Hill, Stoke Newington (1905) and a Reformatory for boys at Wood End Green

Road, Hayes End (1920). All three later became Approved Schools, with the Uxbridge Road establishment moving to Weybridge in 1937.

The Quakers

In 1696, the Society of Friends, or Quakers, established a workhouse-like institution in Bristol for members of the Quaker community. It proved so successful that, in 1700, it moved to purpose-built premises which incorporated an orphanage, a school and an almshouse. Two years later, a workhouse was opened in Clerkenwell for impoverished children and elderly Quakers. By the nineteenth century, the Clerkenwell establishment had become a boarding school for children of Quaker parents who were 'not in affluent circumstances'.[8]

In 1844, a group of Quaker women in Norwich opened an establishment to provide lodgings for female factory workers who had no family to reside with. In 1848, however, the focus changed and it instead housed five orphan or destitute girls who were to be boarded, clothed, educated and trained for domestic service.

At Halstead, in Essex, a Certified Industrial School for Girls was founded in 1869 by Miss Lucy Greenwood, a Quaker, who for some years previously had worked to promote the welfare of the destitute and neglected children in the area. It received financial support from the Quaker community and from friends of Miss Greenwood, including the textile magnate, Samuel Courtald, who had set up a silk mill in Halstead. The School closed in 1921.

In 1943, the Society of Friends opened the Langham Oaks Approved School in Langham, near Colchester, which was in operation until 1956.

Chapter 13

Children with Disabilities

Many early children's homes explicitly denied admission to those with any mental or bodily infirmity. From the end of the eighteenth century, however, institutions caring for children with various forms of disability – blindness, deafness, and physical or mental incapacity – gradually began to appear. In some cases, these establishments admitted adults as well as children. As far as the children were concerned, the usual aim was to provide them with practical skills that would eventually enable them to support themselves.

Blind Children

The earliest charitable institution in England catering specifically for blind children was the School of Instruction for the Indigent Blind, established in Liverpool in 1791, with the blind poet and reformer Edward Rushton usually credited with having originated the idea. The School was subsequently renamed the Asylum for the Indigent Blind. Both titles were somewhat misleading as the establishment offered no residential accommodation and its educational provision was largely confined to training its pupils in a range of trades such as spinning, basket-making and rug-making. Music was also taught and by 1825, fifty-nine of its students were sufficiently competent to have been appointed as church organists.[1]

In the years that followed, a number of broadly similar institutions were founded including Bristol's Asylum for the Blind (1793), Edinburgh's Asylum for the Industrious Blind (1793), London's School for the Indigent Blind (1799) and the Asylum and School for the Indigent Blind in Norwich (1805).

The London establishment, situated in St George's Fields, Southwark, admitted children from the age of 12 upwards, who were clothed, boarded, lodged and instructed. The boys were trained in the production of hampers, wicker baskets, cradles, and rope mats. The girls made fine and coarse thread, window sash-lines and clothes-line. The goods produced were sold to support the charity's funds. Pupils remained at the institution until they had gained a sufficient knowledge of their trade, typically three to four years. It was expected,

however, that children from the poorest backgrounds would only benefit from their training if they had friends able to continue supplying
them with the materials necessary to carry out the trades in which
they had been instructed.[2] The School subsequently occupied extensive premises on Lambeth Road, which it occupied until 1901 when it
moved out to Leatherhead.

Institutions offering a broader education, in addition to purely
vocational training, began to appear in the 1830s. The Yorkshire School
for the Blind, founded in York in 1833, provided 'maintenance, and
ordinary, musical, and industrial instruction for blind children of both
sexes'. Admission was by election and candidates had to be between
the ages of 10 and 16, healthy, capable of learning, and with no more
sight than was sufficient to distinguish light from darkness. An
annual payment of £12 was required, which included clothes. Inmates
remained at the School for seven years. In 1890, Braille's, Moon's and
Roman type were used to teach the pupils reading, and earnings were
said to average 12s. to 14s. a week.[3]

Other establishments of the period included the London Society
for Teaching the Blind to Read (1838), Henshaw's Blind Asylum
in Manchester (1838), the Blind Asylum in Brighton (1839) and the
General Institution for the Blind in Birmingham (1847). The London
Society, now the London Society for Blind People, was founded by
Thomas Lucas who invented an early form of embossed text, known
as Lucas type, which could be read by fingertip touch.

The main provision for Roman Catholics was the Elementary
Education School for Blind Children in Liverpool, founded in 1841. It
offered 'an elementary education and instruction in those branches of
industry which shall be found suitable to each pupil's capacity'.[4]

The College for the Blind Sons of Gentlemen, opened in Worcester
in 1866, was the first higher education establishment for the blind.
Its co-founder, the Reverend William Taylor, invented the Taylor
Arithmetic Frame, a piece of apparatus used to help teach blind students arithmetic using numbers embossed onto movable pegs.

The Elementary Education (Blind and Deaf Children) Act of 1893
made it obligatory for parents to ensure that such children received
a suitable education. In some cases, particularly in major urban areas
such as London, this could be achieved by attendance at a special centre, often attached to an ordinary school. Alternative options offered by
the London School Board included boarding out a child near a suitable
centre, or paying the travelling expenses of an escort guide – usually
a child attending the associated ordinary school.[5] In 1902, the Board

opened two residential schools providing older blind children with vocational training. Elm Court, in Tulse Hill, eventually housed about forty-five girls aged from 12 to 16. As well as ordinary education, half of the working week was spent in the technical teaching of subjects such as chair-caning, basket work, knitting, sewing, rug-making and typewriting. The girls also learned cooking and laundry skills at one of the Board's domestic economy centres. The boys' home, Linden Lodge, in Wandsworth Common, accommodated forty boarders, with basket-making being the main skill taught.

The Royal National Institute for the Blind was founded in 1868 as the British and Foreign Blind Association for Improving the Embossed Literature of the Blind and was influential in the adoption of the Braille alphabet. However, it was not until 1918 that it opened the first of its Sunshine Homes in Chorleywood, Hertfordshire. The home, a residential nursery school, accommodated twenty-five 2-to-5-year-olds whose home conditions were poor. In 1921, the Institute founded Chorleywood College, the first higher education establishment for blind girls, its opening coming sixty-five years after that of the boys' college in Worcester.

Deaf Children

Britain's first school for the deaf was Thomas Braidwood's Academy for the Deaf and Dumb, established in Edinburgh in 1760. It was a rather select establishment, its small number of wealthy pupils being boarded in the founder's own large house. Braidwood is said to have been secretive about his methods, possibly fearing competition from rivals. As well as using traditional techniques such as teaching his pupils to lip-read and to try to learn to speak, he is credited with devising a system of hand gestures, an approach which eventually evolved into the British Sign Language.

In 1783, Braidwood moved to London and opened a school in Hackney, where he was assisted by his nephew, Joseph Watson. In 1792, Watson was appointed as Principal of the newly established Asylum for the Support and Education of the Deaf and Dumb Children of the Poor – the country's first public institution for such children. The Asylum was founded through the efforts of the Reverend John Townsend, a Congregational minister, following a suggestion from a Mrs Creasy, whose son had been a pupil of Braidwood. At its opening, in premises on Grange Road, Bermondsey, the Asylum had six inmates. In 1809, when it moved to the Old Kent Road, the number had risen to seventy.

In 1902, the institution, by now known as the Royal Asylum for Deaf and Dumb Poor, moved to Margate where it became known as the Royal School for Deaf and Dumb Children. The Old Kent Road site was then take over by the London School Board and became a school for 'physically defective' and deaf children.

In 1810, the Edinburgh Institution for the Deaf and Dumb began operation, with Thomas Braidwood's grandson, John, briefly as its headmaster. The Institution admitted children aged from 9 to 14 years, who were certified as having had smallpox.

Two years later, the Institution for the Instruction of the Deaf and Dumb (later known as the Royal Institution for the Instruction of Deaf Children) was established in Edgbaston with another of Thomas Braidwood's grandsons, also named Thomas, appointed as the teacher.

Glasgow's Deaf and Dumb Institution was founded in 1819 by John Anderson and occupied a building in Townhead, on the Barony Glebe. Anderson resigned in 1821 and went off to open a private school in St Andrew's Square.

Further institutions which received deaf children followed in Manchester (1823), Liverpool (1825), Exeter (1826), Doncaster (1829), Newcastle (1838), Brighton (1842) and Aberystwyth (1847). These early establishments were protective places and gave children very limited contact with the outside world. The education they provided was rather basic, and although they offered some practical training, many of their inmates subsequently failed to find employment and ended up destitute.[6]

Two homes were set up for children of particular faiths. In 1863, the Jews' Deaf and Dumb Home was opened in Whitechapel, moving in 1875 to Notting Hill, and in 1899 to Nightingale Lane, Wandsworth. The St John's Institution for Deaf and Dumb Catholic Children was founded in 1870 by a Belgian priest, Canon Désiré de Haerne, and run by the Daughters of Charity of St Vincent de Paul. Its first premises were at Handsworth Woodhouse, near Sheffield, but it moved into a new building in Boston Spa in 1875. Applicants had to be at least 7 years of age, of sound mind and capable of instruction, not liable to fits, and have been vaccinated or had smallpox. In addition to their ordinary education, the boys were taught trades, and the girls learned household work, laundry work, and needlework.

Of the national charities, the Barnardo's Home for Deaf and Dumb Girls, opened in 1900 at 51 Mare Street, Hackney, was the only one at that period which provided facilities for such children. It later became mixed and also added provision for blind and physically disabled children.

From the 1870s, the London School Board established a number of day centres for deaf children. In 1903, it opened a residential home in Anerley, to provide technical training for older boys. A home for girls was opened in 1905 at Oak Lodge, Wandsworth, next door to the Jews' Deaf and Dumb Home. After the Anerley home closed in 1957, Oak Lodge became mixed and continues to provide a residential and day school for students with hearing, speech and communication needs.

In 1900, the London County Council opened its Home for Deaf Children in Homerton, which subsequently became the only such establishment to be certified as an Industrial School. The home moved to Buckinghamshire in 1921 and became known as Rayners School, later acting as the only Approved School for deaf children.

Physical Disability

Residential care for children who were physically disabled – a group commonly referred to as 'cripples' up until the 1960s – was slower to appear than that for those who were deaf or blind and was much more limited in scale. An 1890 directory featured twelve pages of entries for residential institutions for the blind, eleven for the deaf and dumb, but only two for establishments for the physically disabled.[7]

As usual, London was the location of most of the early initiatives, the first being the Female Refuge, founded in 1851 by Mrs Caroline Blount and initially situated at Hill Street, Marylebone. In 1859, the establishment – by then known as the 'Cripples Home' – became a Certified Industrial School, allowing it to receive girls – not necessarily disabled – who had been committed by magistrates. The large majority of the residents were, however, voluntary cases. The girls, aged from 12 upwards, were given lessons in reading and writing by ladies from the home's committee and also received training in straw plaiting, straw hat-making and needlework. The domestic work of the home was performed by the 'industrial' inmates who attended to the wants of the 'cripples' and who also ran a public laundry.

In 1862, a complementary institution, the Cripples' Nursery for Boys and Girls, was established by Lady Victoria Buxton at Henrietta Street, Marylebone. It admitted children between the ages of 3 and 8 and kept them until the age of twelve. A branch of the Nursery was subsequently opened in Margate.

The National Industrial Home for Crippled Boys, located next door to the Kensington workhouse, opened its doors in 1865. Its object was 'to receive for three years – board, and clothe, and educate on Christian principles – destitute, neglected, or ill-used crippled boys, not under 13 years of age nor over 18, and teach them a trade'.[8] In 1870, the home's committee opened a second establishment, the Moore Street Home for Crippled Orphan Boys. Situated just off the Edgware Road, in premises previously occupied by a ragged school, it received boys aged from 8 to 13 who were required to be able to get about on crutches and to dress themselves without assistance. Inmates were taught jewellery- and boot-making.

One of the first institutions outside London was the Home for Crippled Children, opened in the Clifton area of Bristol in 1876. It admitted boys from the ages of 2 to 7 who could remain until the age of 10, while girls were accepted up to the age of 10 and kept until 12 or fourteen. Like others of its type, the home was particular about whom it was prepared to admit. 'Incurable cases of idiocy and epilepsy, and children with any infectious disorder' and 'incurable cases of spine disease and of paralysis of the lower part of the body' were all considered ineligible.[9] Other small, independent homes followed in Abingdon, Berkhamsted and Tiverton.

Care for the physically disabled was one area where the large national charities made a significant contribution, with a number of homes being dedicated to this end. One of the first of these was the St Nicholas' Home for Crippled Children, opened in 1887 by the Waifs and Strays Society in Upper Tooting following a fund-raising campaign for the purpose linked to Queen Victoria's golden jubilee celebrations. In 1893, the home moved to West Byfleet where sixty children could now be accommodated, comprising girls aged from 3 to 12 and boys below the age of seven. Apart from being larger than the old building in Tooting, it had very few stairs which made life much easier for those in wheelchairs. In 1908, the home moved to purpose-built premises in Pyrford, near Woking.

The Society's St Martin's Home for Crippled Boys was opened in Surbiton in 1898, accommodating twenty-one boys aged from 8 to fourteen. In addition to classroom education, the boys were taught tailoring to help improve their prospects for future employment. In 1916, St Martin's moved to Pyrford on a site adjacent to the St Nicholas' Home, the two eventually being amalgamated under the rather cumbersome name of the St Nicholas' and St Martin's Orthopaedic Hospital Homes and Special School of Recovery. The Bradstock Lockett Hospital in Southport, opened in 1908, provided a similar facility serving the north of England. The Society's other major establishment, opened in 1889, was the St Chad's Home in Leeds, where around eighty disabled and 'delicate' girls were occupied in a successful enterprise manufacturing socks and stockings.

Barnardo's first provision was the Jones Memorial Home for 'crippled and incurable children', opened in 1894 in Birkdale, near Southport. The property was donated to the charity in memory of E. H. Jones, a leading figure in the Liverpool branch of the Society for the Prevention of Cruelty to Children. Thomas Barnardo paid great attention to the fitting-out of the home, specifying that the cots had springs and moveable sides. In contrast to the usual practice in Barnardo's homes, boys and girls were allowed to be nursed together.

In 1898, Barnardo opened a Home for Incurables in Bradford, with much of its funding coming from its Young Helpers' League. The Home's twenty-three beds, or rather cots, were allocated to various Yorkshire branches of the League so that supporters could more readily visit those which their own benevolence was supporting. Another Home for Incurables was opened in Tunbridge Wells in 1908.

The National Children's Home's main provision was its home in Chipping Norton, opened in 1903, eventually accommodating a hundred convalescent and physically disabled children. Among its first intake were a victim of severe hemiplegia, a child suffering from spinal curvature and the daughter of an operative killed in a recent catastrophic explosion at the Woolwich Arsenal. As well as training in basket-making and rug-making, the children were encouraged to develop their musical skills in singing and playing instruments such as the violin, dulcimer and mandolin. Later known as the Penhurst School, the home continued in operation until 2013, with John Buchanan, the 'artist without hands', among its former inmates.

Little in the way of special accommodation for the physically disabled was contributed by the Poor Law authorities. A notable exception was Swinton House School of Recovery, opened by the Manchester Union in 1905, which eventually housed up to 120 children.

Three other individuals should be mentioned in connection with disabled young people. The work of the first, John Groom, began in the 1860s, when he became concerned with the situation of blind and disabled girls on the streets around Farringdon Market who scraped a living selling flowers and watercress to passers-by. Groom hired a large meeting room near Covent Garden and founded the 'Watercress and Flower Girls' Christian Mission', where food and washing facilities were provided. He subsequently set up a manufacturing facility at Clerkenwell, where the Girls' Flower Brigade, as they became

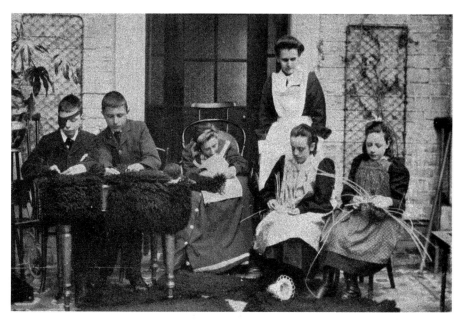

The Waifs and Strays Society's Chipping Norton home, opened in 1903 for 'delicate and affected children'. Inmates with various physical disabilities are making baskets and rugs.

known, produced artificial flowers. In 1894, the operation moved to larger premises on Sekforde Street, with accommodation also being provided as part of what was now called John' Groom's Crippleage. In 1890, Groom also opened a home for orphaned or abandoned children in Clacton, which also provided a holiday venue for the London flower girls.

The second name is that of Grace Kimmins who promoted the use of play in the education of disabled children. After founding the London-based Guild of the Poor Brave Things in 1894, she took over a former workhouse site at Chailey in Sussex and in 1902 established the Heritage Craft School and Hospital for Crippled Children which became a major therapeutic centre.

The third figure of note is Sir William Purdie Treloar who, during his tenure as Lord Mayor of London in 1906–7, raised the sum of £10,000 in his mayoral 'Cripples' Fund'. The money was used to found Lord Mayor Treloar Cripples' Home, Hospital and College on the site of a former war hospital near Alton, Hampshire, which was donated for the purpose by the government. The institution provided a convalescent home for children from orthopaedic and other hospitals who would otherwise be unable to obtain the needed rest and change of air. The hospital department treated children up to the age of 12 who were suffering from tuberculosis of the bones or joints. The college taught technical skills such as leather bag-making to physically disabled boys aged from 14 to eighteen. Lessons for the younger children took place out of doors whenever possible and the facilities in the grounds included a forest school and a large aviary. The hospital section later joined the National Health Service as the Lord Mayor Treloar Orthopaedic Hospital. The college, now based in nearby Holybourne, still provides education and support for disabled young people.

Tuberculosis

An infectious disease rather than a 'disability', tuberculosis (TB or consumption) was the cause of many children spending lengthy periods in institutional care. The incidence of the disease is usually associated with factors such as poverty, poor housing, overcrowding and poor nutrition, and at the end of the nineteenth century it had become Britain's major public health concern. Although TB most often affects the lungs, it can also attack other parts of the body such as the digestive system or the joints and bones, resulting in a progressive weakening and wasting of the body, in some cases leading to permanent physical disability. Prior to the development of antibiotics, the treatments for TB and various forms of physical disability had much in common, namely fresh air, sunshine, physiotherapy and rest. These were usually provided at special-purpose sanatoria, whose designs were characterized by large, open, south-facing balconies onto which beds or trolleys could be wheeled.

Many of the children who came into the care of children's charities suffered from TB and a number of organizations established their own treatment facilities. Barnardo's was first off the mark, with the Edmund Hannay Watts Sanatorium, opened in 1904 at the Girls' Village Home, although prior to this date some treatment was probably provided at Her Majesty's Hospital, opened in 1877 at the Stepney Causeway site. In 1911, the new Australasian Hospital came into operation at the Girls' Village Home and it then dealt with acute TB cases, with the Watts Sanatorium used for less severe and convalescent cases.

In 1904, the Waifs and Strays Society opened a seaside convalescent home in Hurstpierpoint in Sussex, with recovering TB patients among its residents. In 1908, the new St Nicholas Home in Pyrford became the

Society's main facility for providing care for the disabled and for TB cases.

In 1908, the Father Hudson's home in Coleshill opened a temporary infirmary to deal with TB cases. It was followed in 1913 by a permanent establishment, St Gerard's Hospital, serving all the Catholic children's homes in the Birmingham diocese and also Catholic children from workhouse infirmaries.

In 1910, the National Children's Home opened the Elmfield Sanatorium in Harpenden, close to its large cottage homes site. Elmfield had sixty-four places for patients aged from 7 to 14 years. The south-facing building had large balconies on which patients could be placed. There was also an open-air school, revolving chalets, covered playgrounds, playing fields, gardens and an open-air rest room. In 1955, Elmfield was converted to serve as a residential school for disabled children.

The Metropolitan Asylums Board (MAB) was formed in 1867 to administer care for certain categories of the sick poor in the capital. It opened two establishments catering for London children with TB. The first, East Cliff House in Margate, was opened in 1898 and specialized in the treatment of tubercular disease of the joints, spine and glands. After the buildings were enlarged in 1919 it re-opened as Princess Mary's Hospital for Children. The second, opened in 1904, was the purpose-built 120-bed Millfield Sanatorium in Rustington, in West Sussex. It was intended for early cases of pulmonary tuberculosis and was the only Poor Law establishment in the country specializing in the treatment of this condition.[10]

Mental Deficiency

As with physical disability, dedicated residential care for children with what would now usually be referred to as severe learning difficulties was slow to appear. Such children were then labelled as 'mentally defective', a term that gradually came to be replaced by expressions such as 'mentally deficient',' mentally subnormal' or 'mentally handicapped'. Three categories of impairment were commonly distinguished. In increasing order of severity these were 'feeble-minded', 'imbecile' and 'idiot', although the exact interpretation of these terms varied. Up until the mid-nineteenth century, the only institutional care available for such conditions was either in a workhouse or an asylum for the mentally ill.

In 1847, Mrs Ann Serea Plumbe, the mother of a mentally handicapped boy, Andrew Reed Plumbe, launched a campaign for the creation of an institution where such children could receive education and training. The cause was taken up by the Reverend Dr Andrew Reed, who had previously founded the London Orphan Asylum and several other important institutions. As a result, the Asylum for Idiots – 'for the care and education of the idiot, especially in the earlier periods of life' – was inaugurated later the same year. In 1848, the Asylum moved into Park House, Highgate, and received its first inmates – thirty boys, including Andrew Reed Plumbe, and three girls. The establishment soon became full and in 1850 an annexe was opened at Essex Hall, a former hotel in Colchester. In the same year, Queen Victoria donated the sum of 250 guineas, constituting the Prince of Wales as life patron and able to appoint to one bed in perpetuity.

Growing pressure on space at the Highgate and Colchester premises led to a public appeal for funds to erect a new 'Asylum for the suitable and permanent reception of the Idiot and Imbecile' on a site in Earlswood, near Redhill, in Surrey. The completed building, with accommodation for 400, was opened in July 1855 by Prince Albert. The addition of new wings in 1873 increased the accommodation to 800 places. Admission to Earlswood was normally by election of the charity's subscribers, and for a period of five years, although paying inmates were also accepted. Inmates were trained in skills such as brush-making, shoe-making, carpentry and printing, or could work in the institution's kitchens and laundry, or on its own farm and market gardens. Known as the Royal Earlswood Asylum from 1862, and later as the Royal Earlswood Hospital, the establishment finally closed in 1997.

Other institutions following the model established at Earlswood included the Eastern Counties Asylum for Idiots and Imbeciles (previously Essex Hall) in Colchester (1859), the Western Counties Idiot Asylum in Starcross, near Exeter (1864), the Royal Albert Asylum in Lancaster (1864) and the Midland Counties Idiot Asylum in Knowle, near Solihull (1868).

Scotland's first institution for the care and education of 'imbecile' children was opened in 1852 in Baldovan, near Dundee. The establishment was part orphanage, with the aim that the imbecile children would benefit from playing with the orphans. In 1863, the Scottish National Institution for the Education of Imbecile Children was opened in Larbert, near Stirling. It was originally intended for children aged between 6 and 12, but the age range was soon expanded.

One of the MAB's earliest projects was the creation of two Imbeciles' Asylums, one located in Leavesden, near Watford, the other in Caterham in Surrey. These institutions, both opened in 1870, each accommodated over 1,500 inmates, a mixture of adults and children. A visitor to a children's ward at Caterham in 1872 found it:

> *lamentable to see so many poor children (fully sixty in number) con-*
> *demned to pass their life within the walls of an asylum ... Their*
> *condition was possibly more to be deplored than that of the adults,*
> *because no healthy occupation could be found for them ... they had a*
> *listless appearance which was exceedingly depressing.*[11]

In 1873, the children from Caterham and Leavesden were transferred to temporary accommodation in Hampstead and teachers appointed in an experiment to try educating 'idiot' children. In 1878, the MAB opened a new institution in Darenth, Kent, for 560 imbecile children aged from 5 to sixteen. 'Improvable' inmates were given workshop training, while the more severely afflicted 'hopeless' were placed in a separate part of the building. In 1911, the MAB's Fountain Hospital in Tooting was converted from a fever hospital into children's accommodation for 'unimprovable imbeciles'.

Special provision for children with mental disability by the major charities was rather limited. Thomas Barnardo believed that it was best for such children to be integrated among their peers rather than placed in special institutions. At the Girls' Village Home, three cottages were eventually allocated for housing the most severe cases, while those less afflicted were distributed around the site. It was found that embroidery could be successfully taught to girls classed as feeble-minded and in 1903 a training school was constructed at the Home. By 1906, fifty girls could support themselves in embroidery, knitting and lace-making. At the same date it was reported that the number of feeble-minded children in the charity's homes was nearly two hundred.[12] In 1912, Barnardo's decided to exclude mentally deficient children from its homes but subsequently relented and from the late 1920s set up or converted several homes to cater for 'backward' children, such as the Howard House home in Bedford, where the novelist and playwright Frank Norman was an inmate for a while.

In 1899, the Elementary Education (Defective and Epileptic Children) Act encouraged local School Boards to provide special facilities for such children from the age of 7 upwards. The London School Board was particularly active in this area and, by 1903, had sixty-one centres for mentally defective children.[13]

Section 62 of the 1908 Children Act allowed institutions catering for various categories of 'mental or physical defect' to be certified as

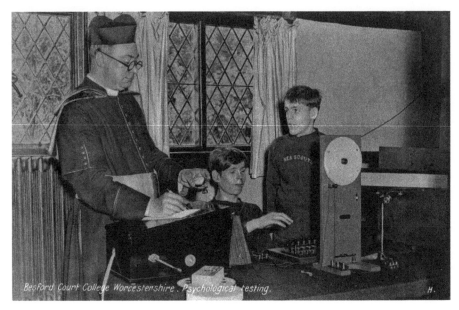

A member of staff carries out psychological testing of two inmates at the Besford Court home for 'high grade mentally defective' Roman Catholic boys.

special Industrial Schools. Around thirty institutions were eventually accredited for this purpose, among the first being the Homerton Residential School for Deaf Children, Hackney and the Stoke Park Colony for Mentally Defective Children, Bristol. Those for Roman Catholic children included Besford Court Colony and Farm School in Worcestershire, and the Pontville School, near Ormskirk, both of which later became Approved Schools for 'high-grade' mental defectives.

In the early 1900s, there was increasing pressure from supporters of the eugenics movement for the feeble-minded to be discouraged or prevented from reproducing. In response to this, the 1913 Mental Deficiency Act gave local authorities the primary responsibility for identifying 'defectives' and providing institutions for their care. Although some local authorities established their own accommodation for this purpose, such as the Meanwood Park Colony opened in 1920 by Leeds Council, most of it was provided by the voluntary sector or the Poor Law authorities. The majority of institutions were either for adults only, or for all ages, but a few focused on children, notably the Sandlebridge Colony in Great Warford, Cheshire, founded in 1902 by the Lancashire and Cheshire Society for the Permanent Care of the Feeble-Minded. The Society's Secretary, Mary Dendy, was influential in promoting the idea that the care of the mentally deficient should be different from that provided for the mentally ill. The 'colony' approach that she promoted – borrowed from the children's cottage homes model – placed inmates in a self-contained community, usually located in an isolated rural area. The advantages of such permanent segregation, according to Dendy, included the prevention of the many crimes supposedly committed by the feeble-minded, a reduction in the overcrowding of workhouses and prisons, which she believed they filled, and the avoidance of the mentally defective being able to pass on their condition to a future generation. It was not until the 1930s that there was gradual acceptance for the view that 'community care was in many cases not only cheaper and more practicable, but better for the patient'.[14] By the 1920s, the Manchester Union's Swinton House home, originally opened to accommodate the physically disabled, had begun to house children with mental difficulties.

Following the death of its founder in 1933, the Waifs and Strays Society launched the Rudolf Memorial Appeal to raise money for two new homes specializing in the care of children with learning difficulties or behavioural problems. Being an area where the Society lacked experience, the homes were run in association with the London Child Guidance Clinic.

In 1952, the NCH's Edgworth home was converted to accommodate children with learning difficulties. The charity's home at Bramhope followed suit in 1957.

A good number of the large old institutions set up to house the mentally deficient were to linger for very many years, with some becoming part of the National Health Service at its inauguration in 1948. In 1974, it was estimated that 7,000 children lived in hospitals for the mentally handicapped due to factors such as shortages of day care, social workers and special schools.[15] The early 1970s also witnessed a number of scandals concerning the neglect and mistreatment of inmates at a number of institutions, including Bristol's Stoke Park Hospital where even its Medical Superintendent described its conditions as slum-like.[16] Despite improvements being made at the site, and the national drive towards care in the community, culminating in the 1990 National Health Service and Community Care Act, Stoke Park did not finally close its doors until 1997.

Epilepsy

Children suffering from epilepsy were usually refused admission to residential care institutions. An early exception to this was the Hospital and Home for Incurable Children, established in 1875 in London's Maida Vale. Children could remain there until the age of 16, at which time they were returned to their family or friends.

In 1888, the first of several residential 'colonies' for epileptics was founded in Maghull, near Liverpool, although the great majority of its inmates were above school age.[17] Five years later, in 1893, Lady Meath founded the Meath Home of Comfort for epileptic girls and women. The institution, in Godalming in Surrey, could accommodate 97 patients who were charged from eight shillings to three guineas a week. Many of the cases were placed by boards of guardians, with the Girls' Friendly Society also subscribing to several beds. Patients who were 'violent, hysterical, imbecile or lunacy cases' were not admitted. The inmates were engaged in occupations such as needlework, beadwork, basket-making or laundry work.[18]

In 1894, the first colony in England for 'sane' epileptics was founded by the National Society for the Employment of Epileptics, in Chalfont St Peter in Buckinghamshire. Applicants for admission were carefully screened to exclude cases of mental deficiency and those who 'by reason of awkwardness, irritability or physical defect' would not be suited to colony life.[19] The original colony buildings included provision for a Certified School but this had to be abandoned and children were not admitted until 1909, after two homes and a school had been built, funded by the local education authority. The number of residents at Chalfont reached a peak of 575 in 1942, around a hundred of those being children.

The first colony specifically for epileptic children was set up in 1897 at Lingfield in Surrey by the Christian Social Service Union. By the 1930s, the site had accommodation for 465 'educable' children aged from 5 upwards. The establishment eventually evolved into what is now the National Centre for Young People with Epilepsy. In 1902, the same organization opened a school and farm colony for epileptic boys in Starnthwaite, near Kendal. The forty inmates, aged from 7 to 16, were given training in carpentry, boot- and shoe-making, rug- and carpet-making, and farm and garden work.

Other provision for children with epilepsy included St Elizabeth's School for Roman Catholic Epileptic Children in Much Hadham, Hertfordshire (1903), the David Lewis Colony for Epileptics in Great Warford, Cheshire (1904), and the House of Mercy adjacent to the Quarrier's Homes in Renfrewshire (1901). In 1917, the Metropolitan Asylums Board began to make provision for juvenile and adult epileptics from the capital. It established a colony for males in the former

Strand Union school in Edmonton and a home for females in a former Hackney Union school in Brentwood, each housing up to 300 inmates. Both were taken over by the London County Council in 1930, respectively becoming the St David's and St Faith's Hospitals.

Other Medical Conditions

Until the middle of the nineteenth century, childhood mortality was generally viewed as unavoidable and hospital provision for children was virtually non-existent. In 1842, of the 2,363 individuals then resident in London's hospitals, only 26 were young children.[20] England's first hospital for children was founded in 1852 in Great Ormond Street, London. The idea was soon taken up across the country, with thirty-eight children's hospitals in operation by 1888.[21]

As well as these general institutions, a few establishments were set up for the treatment of particular conditions. Two infectious diseases which were especially common among children living in overcrowded or insanitary conditions were ringworm (a fungal infection affecting the scalp, body, feet and nails) and ophthalmia (an inflammatory condition of the eye). In 1899, the Home for Children Suffering from Ringworm was opened in West Horsley, Surrey, and accredited as a Certified School. Two years later, the MAB opened a 400-bed residential treatment centre for ringworm in the former workhouse in Witham in Essex, followed in 1903 by a similar facility in Sutton in Surrey. The introduction of X-ray treatment for ringworm in 1905 led to a much speedier cure for the condition.

In 1903–4, the MAB established two residential treatment centres for ophthalmia – White Oak School in Swanley in Kent, and High Wood School in Brentwood in Essex, both cottage homes developments, each housing 360 children. In 1910, the St John Baptist Home for the treatment of ophthalmia among Roman Catholic boys was opened in Chigwell, with the St Anne's Home for Catholic girls being opened in Notting Hill. St Margaret's Hospital in Kentish Town was opened by the MAB in 1917 for the treatment of ophthalmia neonatorum, a form of conjunctivitis mostly commonly contracted during delivery by an infant whose mother is infected with gonorrhoea.

Chapter 14

Fund Raising

As well as the basic business of looking after the children in their care, the biggest concern of most voluntary institutions was the ongoing raising of funds to support that work. The financial situation of many organizations was often precarious, with some of the larger charities burdened by long-term debts running into thousands of pounds.

As well as collecting one-off donations, charities were always keen to recruit annual subscribers to provide a regular source of income from year to year. Recognition could be given to donors and subscribers in various ways, such as the publication of their names and gifts in a charity's annual reports or even in local newspapers. In some cases, contributions above a certain amount could earn the giver the right to vote in the election of new entrants to the organization's institutions. Another possible perk was attendance at social events such as annual dinners or other meetings where a charity's patron might be present. As many charities discovered, the support of a distinguished person such as a member of the nobility, or even of the royal family, could substantially benefit its income. The Orphan Working School at Hampstead was particularly successful in its endeavours. As well as having Queen Victoria as its patron, it could count eminent individuals such as Charles Dickens among its donors, with its corporate subscribers including the Corporation of London and more than twenty City Livery Companies.

Legacies (gifts of cash) and bequests (gifts of property or other possessions) formed another valuable source of income. In 1885, a £25,000 legacy from Mr Thomas Wheeler, of Rock, near Bewdley, enabled major extensions to be made to Worcester's Royal Albert Orphanage, together with the purchase of an additional six acres of land. The Jones Memorial Home for 'crippled and incurable children' was opened in 1894 at Birkdale, near Southport, on a property bequeathed to Barnardo's in memory of E. H. Jones, a leading figure in the Society for the Prevention of Cruelty to Children in the area. In 1918, the former Penarth Hotel on Paget Place, Penarth, was donated to the NCH by the Gibbs family in memory of Major J. A. Gibbs, who had died in the First World War. As the J. A. Gibbs Memorial Home, it educated and trained boys for naval service.

Another popular form of financial support for an institution was by naming a bed or cot at the establishment. This could be by an individual, a society, a school or other organization. As well as an initial donation, typically £50, the giving of a subsequent annual 'maintenance fee' was also encouraged. The name, coat of arms or emblem of the donor was usually commemorated either by hanging a brass plaque on the bed or by a smaller plate attached to the frame of a suitable picture hung above it.

Most charities undertook an ongoing programme of fund-raising activities to finance the running costs of their work. This included advertisements in newspapers and magazines, and also 'letters to the editor' to commend the work of an organization or institution and invite support.

In 1894, Barnardo launched Self-Denial Week, during which supporters were encouraged to forego unnecessary comforts. For example, families could consume only the plainest of foods, children could give up sweets, and businessmen could travel third class. The accumulated savings over the week could then be given to the charity. The scheme was soon raising several thousands of pounds each year.[1]

Also in 1894, Barnardo inaugurated an annual street collection. 'Waif Saturday', modelled on the already established 'Hospital Saturday', featured an army of women who were each provided with a distinctive collecting box, armband, literature and authorization card. The collectors were under the protective watch of uniformed Barnardo

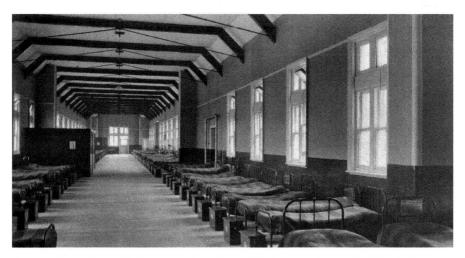

A dormitory at the Wolverhampton Royal Orphanage. Several of the beds carry brass plaques memorializing their endowment.

boys or local police. In 1898, Barnardo boasted that one of his collectors had successfully accosted the Prince of Wales for a donation.[2] The following year, house-to-house leafleting, with a follow-up call for donations, proved even more successful. Other charities gradually followed suit. In 1901–2, the NCH received a total of £61 from street collections, more than half of which was from a single town – Cambridge. In 1940, the Home's income from street and house-to-house collections had risen to £54,000.[3]

From the late 1880s, the Waifs and Strays Society's Children's Union involved young people in its fund-raising efforts through the sale of small articles they had made. In 1897, ten years after its founding, the Union's 8,843 members raised a total of £2,820.[4] Thomas Barnardo adopted a similar strategy with the formation in 1891 of the Young Helpers' League. In 1892, the League's income was £2,186 and in 1906, the year after Barnardo's death, raised £18,505.[5] The NCH launched its own scheme in 1899 with the founding of the Young Leaguer's Union. Other NCH fund-raisers included its Birthday Society, which encouraged members to send a donation to the Home on their birthday,

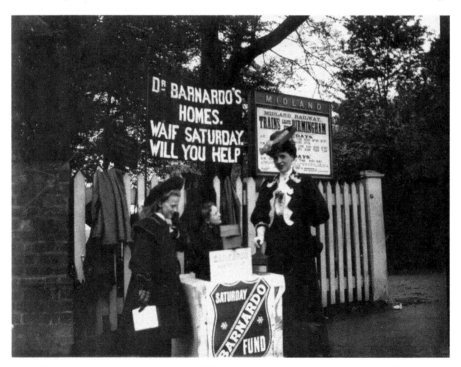

A well-dressed woman and two children run a collection point on Barnardo's 'Waif Saturday' in 1906.

and its Order of St Christopher – 'a fellowship of individual workers for child welfare'. In 1900, the Shaftesbury Homes encouraged donations by children from comfortable homes through its 'Victoria League' for girls, and 'Arethusa League' for boys.

Not long after Barnardo's death, a former member of his Young Helper's League proposed a scheme to encourage regular small-scale donations from the poor, based on a contribution of a farthing a week. The National Farthing League, as it was named, was hugely successful, with its annual income reaching £33,000 by the end of the First World War. In the 1920s, the Waifs and Strays Society provided supporters with Penny Boxes into which a penny a week could be deposited over the course of a year. With an extra top-up at Christmas, this would amount to ten shillings – about the weekly cost of maintaining a child in one of the Society's homes.

The children's homes themselves could become involved in fund-raising efforts. In the 1890s, the Pound Day became a popular annual event, with supporters of a particular home invited to contribute a pound weight of some useful household commodity such as flour, sugar, rice or tea. Alternatively, the gift could consist of silver or copper coins weighing a pound or to the value of a pound. Income could also be generated by the sale of goods produced by the children at the home, such as items knitted, sewn or embroidered by the girls. These would typically be sold at one of periodic bazaars or other events run by friends of the establishment. The St Chad's Home in Leeds, for physically disabled or 'delicate' girls, specialized in the manufacture of high-quality socks and stockings which were sold by mail order.

One of Barnardo's major annual events was its Founder's Day celebration held at the Girls' Village Home at Barkingside. In 1935, the occasion was attended by the Duke and Duchess of York and featured contributions from various Barnardo establishments, such as gymnastic, musical marching and field-gun displays, boys' and Brownies' bands and maypole, hornpipe and sword dancing. Art embroidery by the girls, and flowers, fruit and vegetables grown by the boys could also be purchased. According to the programme for the event (price 6d.) visitors were invited to contribute a half-crown to the £400,000 required to feed all the charity's children each year.[6]

Musical performances by the children were often used to assist fund-raising. Many boys' establishments had a military-style wind band which could be engaged for performances at fêtes or other events. Barnardo particularly encouraged musical training among the inmates of his Stepney Causeway home. His 'musical boys' could turn their hands to a wide range of instruments including mandolins, guitars, xylophones, dulcimers, hand-bells, sleigh bells, ocarinas, cornets and bagpipes, and groups travelled around the country to perform at fund-raising events. In 1891, eight of the boys accompanied the Reverend Walter Mayers on a trip to Australia where £10,000 was raised for Barnardo funds. A similar party visited Australia and New Zealand in 1908 and raised almost £17,500 which was used for the construction of the Australian Hospital at the Girls' Village Home.

St Hilda's – the Waifs and Strays Society's home for girls in Bradford, West Yorkshire – developed a strong musical tradition after a percussion band was started in 1936. It was instigated by Mr Stephen Moore, the Honorary Secretary of the Worcestershire Association of Musical Societies, who had encountered the home while visiting Bradford on other business. The following year, the band played on the radio as part of a talk given by Mr Moore. They also appeared on two gramophone records and were even visited by Sir Adrian Boult who listened to them playing along with some of his own orchestral recordings.

Singers, too, made a contribution. A band of choirboys and hand-bell ringers from Spurgeon's Home at Stockwell regularly gave performances over a wide area. The choir at the NCH home in Harpenden was very well regarded, as were those at the Shaftesbury Home in Twickenham and at Josiah Mason's Orphanage in Birmingham, the latter being regularly featured in BBC radio broadcasts in the 1920s and '30s.

Some of the larger charities, such as Barnardo's and the Waifs and Strays Society, offered 'an evening with the children' through the hiring out of sets of lantern slides, with a hire fee or audience collection resulting in a donation to the organization.

From the 1930s, the cinema began to join the list of media through which children's charities could keep themselves in the public eye. Homes occasionally featured in the newsreels produced by Movietone and British Pathé, such as on the occasion of a royal visit. The NCH was one of the first charities to actively exploit the cinema with the production of specially filmed appeals such as *The Seven Lamps* featuring Sybil Thorndike, and *Broken Wings* with the actor Leslie Banks.[7]

Competition between charities for the public's support was often intense. Appeal leaflets and advertisements were invariably packed with impressive statistics enumerating how many homes were run by the organization, how many children it had in its care, and so on.

The level of donations could fluctuate according to the state of the economy, with downturns occurring particularly in wartime.

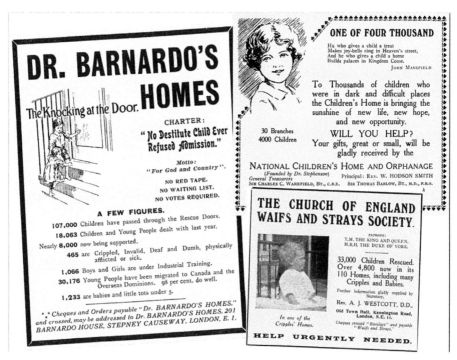

Fund-raising advertisements from the 'big three' charities in around 1930.

Inevitably, over the years, some charities failed to raise enough funds to keep going and were forced to close down or merge with other organizations. In 1920, just seven years short of its centenary, this was the fate of the British Orphan Asylum whose financial difficulties forced it to shut its doors and amalgamate with the London Orphan Asylum.

Chapter 15

Poor Law Homes

As already noted, some of the earliest institutional accommodation for homeless or destitute children was provided by the Poor Law authorities in cities such as London and Bristol. This was a role that workhouses and their associated establishments were to continue performing until well into the twentieth century.

The Old Poor Law

The Poor Relief Act of 1601, the foundation of what became known as the Old Poor Law, made the parish the focus of the administration of poor relief, funded by a local property tax known as the poor rate. Those in need were primarily helped by means of 'out relief' – hand-outs – which might be in cash or in kind. The 1601 Act made relatively little mention of pauper children except to say that they were to be put to work or apprenticed. The Act also made no reference to the workhouse, an institution that gradually developed over the following century or so, as a convenient method for accommodating the 'blameless' poor – the elderly, chronic sick, disabled and so on. The workhouse also provided a place where the able-bodied poor could be given board and lodging in return for performing labour – a test of their destitution.

Early workhouses were set up in towns such as Reading and Sheffield (1628), Leeds (1638) and by the City of London (1648). At the end of the seventeenth century, larger towns began to obtain their own local parliamentary Acts enabling them to manage poor relief at a town rather than a parish level and to raise money specifically to finance the running of a large workhouse. From the 1720s, parishes were able to discourage claims for poor relief by making the workhouse the only option on offer, at least for those who were able-bodied. This, coupled with the advent of 'farming the poor' – the running of workhouses by private contractors – could reduce the cost to a parish of relieving its poor, thus making the setting-up of a workhouse an attractive money-saving proposition. By the 1770s, around one in seven parishes had gone down this path, with almost 2,000 workhouses then operating in England and Wales.[1]

Children formed just another part of the very mixed population to be found living in the parish workhouses of the day, which could also include the elderly, the disabled, single mothers and their children, and the mentally ill or incapacitated. Although some provided their child inmates with a little basic education and training in crafts such as spinning and weaving, the management of many workhouses was one of benign neglect.

For some children, an escape from the workhouse was provided by apprenticeship. From around the age of 10, a parish could place a child – together with a premium, typically of £5 – with a tradesman or other employer, who would train, clothe and maintain it until at least the age of eighteen. From the late eighteenth century until the 1830s, the boom in large-scale textile manufacture saw many workhouse children being sent as apprentices to work in cotton and woollen mills in the north of England, sometimes from as far away as London. Some employers built special accommodation for their armies of child workers. At the Quarry Bank mill in Styal, Cheshire, the Apprentice House became the long-term home for sixty girls and thirty boys.

Baby Farms

In 1766, the unhealthy conditions which then existed in many London workhouses prompted the passing of Jonas Hanway's Act. This demanded that all pauper children from metropolitan parishes were to reside at least three miles from the capital until they attained the age of six. The nursing and maintenance of each child was to cost at least 2s. 6d. per week.

To satisfy these requirements, parishes sent their children to a variety of out-of-town establishments, sometimes known as 'infant poorhouses' or 'baby farms', many of which were privately run. For example, infants from the parish of St Luke were put out to nurse at Southgate where an average of fifty children were under the care of three nurses. Shoreditch had its own establishment at Baker Street in Enfield, with a resident master, matron and 'suitable assistants'. St George's, Southwark, had an infant poorhouse which stood opposite Lewisham's workhouse, while that used by Islington was in Fords Green, Lower Edmonton. Other establishments were located in Hendon (used by St Clement Danes), Merton (St Mary Magdalen, Bermondsey), Heston (St Giles in the Fields and St George, Bloomsbury) and Barnet (St Andrew Holborn and St George the Martyr). Two of the largest institutions were Mr Aubin's school in Norwood and Mr Drouet's school in Tooting, each of which served a number of London's parishes.

The New Poor Law

Despite the rise of the workhouse, out relief always remained the dominant means by which parishes relieved their poor. In 1832, in an effort to stem its ever rising cost, a Royal Commission was appointed to conduct a complete review of the administration of poor relief. Two years later, recommendations in the Commission's report resulted in the 1834 Poor Law Amendment Act, which became known as the New Poor Law.

The new system was organized around groupings of parishes known as Poor Law unions, usually centred on a town in each area. Each union was locally administered by a board of guardians, a committee elected by the ratepayers in each member parish, with the financing of poor relief continuing to come from the household poor rate. Each union was expected to provide a large and strictly run workhouse to serve its whole area. The New Poor Law aimed to put an end to out relief for the able-bodied poor and make the workhouse the only option on offer. A central body known as the Poor Law Commissioners (PLC) supervised the new system from their headquarters at Somerset House in London.

Union Workhouses

One distinctive, and much-hated, feature of the new union workhouses was their strict segregation of different classes of inmate – male and female, the elderly and the able-bodied, and children. Families were split up, with fathers being placed in the men's section and mothers in the women's quarters. Boys aged from 7 to 14 had their own area, as did the girls. Children under 7 were allowed to live in the women's wards, with many workhouses operating some kind of nursery to provide care for the younger children while their mothers worked. Such provision was often very basic – little more than a bare room supervised by an elderly female inmate.

Parents having children in the same workhouse could request a supervised daily 'interview' with their offspring. In practice, more informal meetings with one or other parent (though not both at the same time) were usually arranged to take place on Sunday afternoons. If children and parents were housed in different establishments, such reunions might be much less frequent.

Although the normal requirement was for whole families to enter the workhouse together or to leave together, there were occasional exceptions to this. Unions sometimes made ad hoc arrangements with families, or even husbandless women, to take one or two of their children – usually the younger ones – into the workhouse if this allowed the rest of the family to continue living independently.

Despite the impression given by Dickens's *Oliver* Twist, the diet of workhouse children did not consist entirely of meagre portions of gruel. Although some of the weekly menu plans issued by the PLC in 1835 did feature gruel or porridge, they also included bread and cheese, suet pudding, soup or broth, with meat dinners several times a week.[2] Children aged 9 or above were allocated the same rations as adult females, while the younger ones were to be fed 'at discretion' – typically bread and milk for breakfast and supper, and an appropriately sized portion of the adult dinner.

As regards discipline, the regulations regarding the punishment of workhouse children were extensive. The use of corporal punishment, or flogging, was restricted to boys who were under the age of 14, and could only be carried out by the schoolmaster or the workhouse master. Two hours had to have elapsed since the offence and the rod used had to have been approved by the board of guardians. The workhouse's refractory cell, used to confine inmates committing more serious infringements of the institution's rules, could not be employed for children under 12 either during the night or if it had no windows.[3]

The education of workhouse children was required to include at least three hours a day of 'reading, writing, arithmetic, and the principles of the Christian religion, and such other instruction shall be imparted to them as may fit them for service, and train them to habits of usefulness, industry, and virtue'.[4] Despite this requirement, boards of guardians were sometimes reluctant to spend money on even the most basic equipment such as writing slates. Some even questioned whether pauper children actually needed to be taught basic literacy. This was partly justified by the 1834 Act's principle of 'less eligibility' – that workhouse conditions would always be less amenable than those outside, even for the poorest independent labourer. This, it was argued, demanded a lower quality of education for children in the workhouse than would be enjoyed by those of modest means outside the workhouse. In 1836, the guardians of the Bedford Union suggested a compromise by teaching workhouse children to read but not to write. Likewise, in 1839 the guardians of the Pershore Union decided that it was 'quite unnecessary to teach the children in the union workhouse the accomplishment of writing'.[5] Those holding such views were eventually persuaded that teaching pauper children to read and write would, in the long run, make them less likely to need poor relief.

Although the majority of union workhouses had their own school-rooms, the increasing trend in the latter half of the nineteenth century was to send children out to local schools. Initially, this would generally have been to one of the National or British Schools that existed in many towns, and then, from 1870, to one of the many Board Schools that were established. Workhouse children, usually being easily identifiable by their clothing, boots or short haircuts, did not always have an easy time and were often stigmatized by their classmates.

In common with other types of children's institution, the idea of 'industrial training' was taken up in New Poor Law workhouses. As with education, the hope of the workhouse administrators was that children with practical skills would be employable in their adult life and therefore much less likely to end up in need of poor relief.

District and Separate Schools

One of the earliest proposals for housing pauper children in separate accommodation away from the union workhouse was for the establishment of District Schools, a scheme first outlined in 1838 by Dr James Kay (later better known as Sir James Kay-Shuttleworth). Kay envisaged that each District School would serve a group of unions, perhaps with an existing workhouse in the area being converted for the purpose.

Kay argued that such establishments would allow children to receive a much better education, together with good industrial training facilities. Kay also believed that such schools would protect pauper children from what he saw as the 'polluting association' with the adult workhouse inmates.[6]

Kay was particularly influenced by Mr Aubin's school in Norwood, which at that time had over 1,000 residential pupils, largely taken from metropolitan Poor Law authorities. After the introduction of industrial training at the school, together with the banning of corporal punishment and improved conditions for teachers, great improvements had taken place in the children's performance and morale. As a result, the school became a much trumpeted showpiece of public education. Kay proposed a grandiose scheme for establishing 100 similar District Schools across England and Wales, each accommodating around 500 children.[7]

Another influential model was the Bridgnorth Union's school in the Shropshire village of Quatt. The school, which accommodated around eighty children, was set up in a large house on the estate owned by

Bridgnorth Union guardian Mr Wolrych Whitmore. As well as receiving a basic classroom education, the boys cultivated the land and managed farm stock, while the girls did the housework.

Although Kay's emphasis on industrial training was widely taken up, it was often on a small scale within existing workhouses and the provision of separate institutions for children was slow to happen. A few large establishments were established in the 1840s by Poor Law authorities in the north of England such as the Manchester Union's Industrial School at Swinton, the Liverpool Vestry's Kirkdale Industrial School, and the Leeds Moral and Industrial Training School. (Despite the similarity in name, these Poor Law Industrial Schools were quite separate from the system of Certified Industrial Schools introduced in 1857.) Separate schools for workhouse children were also established by individual unions in Brighton, Cardiff, Chesterfield, Cockermouth, Halstead, Hartismere, Merthyr Tydfil and Oxford.

Kay's proposals for the establishment of District Schools were incorporated into the 1844 Poor Law Amendment Act, allowing unions within a fifteen-mile radius (later extended to twenty miles) to form a School District for the purposes of setting up joint schools. The anticipated benefits of the larger District Schools included economies of scale in teaching larger classes, the ability to provide industrial

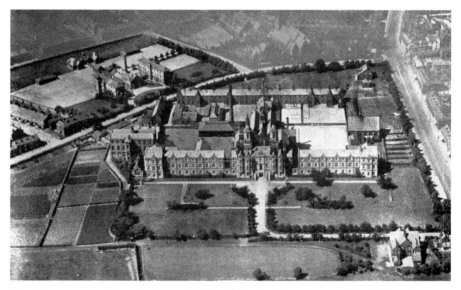

The Manchester Union Industrial Schools in Swinton, opened in 1845, where up to 800 pauper children were housed. At the top left is the Union's Swinton House home for disabled children, opened in 1905.

training in a wider range of subjects than a single workhouse could offer; savings in the cost of staff, furniture, books etc., and the provision of better-quality staff who would be attracted to such establishments. Despite much encouragement by the central authorities, the scheme never took off, particularly outside London where only four School Districts were ever created: Reading & Wokingham (1849), Farnham & Hartley Wintney (1849), South East Shropshire (1849) and Walsall & West Bromwich (1869).

In the capital, three School Districts were formed in 1849 (Central London, South Metropolitan and North Surrey) which covered ten of the capital's thirty Poor Law authorities. However, a severe blow to the image of large pauper schools occurred in the same year when an outbreak of cholera at Mr Drouet's School in Tooting resulted in the deaths of 180 of its 1,400 resident children. Despite ongoing efforts by the Poor Law Board, it was not until 1868 that three further School Districts (Forest Gate, West London and Finsbury) were created, although Finsbury was dissolved the following year. The Kensington & Chelsea School District was established in 1876, followed by Brentwood in 1877, the latter being dissolved in 1885. By the 1890s, London had five District Schools in operation covering fifteen unions, together with eleven individual separate schools in Bethnal Green, St George-in-the-East, Hackney, Holborn, Islington, Lambeth, St Marylebone, Mile End, St Pancras, Strand and Westminster. Two metropolitan parishes – Hampstead and Bloomsbury St Giles – had no schools of their own, with Hampstead sending its children to the Westminster Union's school in Tooting, and St Giles to the Strand Union's Millfield School in Edmonton.

The Central London District Schools, in Hanwell, was one of the largest of these institutions – in 1881 there were over 1,200 inmates aged from 3 upwards. The activities of the children were organized in two 'divisions' – the working division and the school division. Up to the age of 9, children stayed in the school division and thereafter spent alternate days in each division. In the school division, they received basic education in literacy and numeracy, with the older boys being taught history, geography and science. In the working division, the children were divided into groups to learn and perform various occupations. For the boys these included tailoring, shoemaking, cleaning, farming and gardening, painting and glazing, carpentry, blacksmithing, and baking. The girls were occupied in needlework, cleaning and attending the dormitories, nursery-maid work, cooking, scullery and dairy work. From the age of 14, boys were sent to their own homes, to

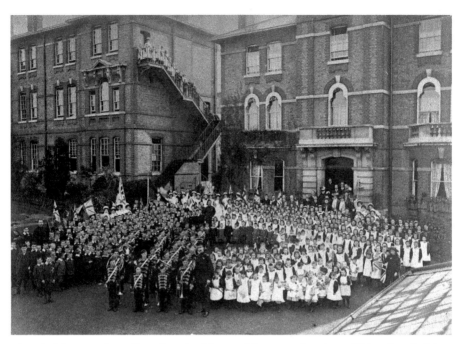

The children and staff at Lambeth's workhouse school on Elder Road, West Norwood. The uniformed boys' band stands at the centre.

working boys' homes, or placed as apprentices. The older girls were given cookery lessons by a qualified teacher and the matron gave special training to those intending to enter domestic service. All the children performed physical drill to provide both exercise and discipline. Boys were taught to play musical instruments and as early as 1865 the School's brass band accompanied mealtimes. Many boys went on to join army bands, several becoming bandmasters.

In 1896, the future film star Charlie Chaplin began a year-long stay at Hanwell. He later recounted the regular Friday morning punishment sessions in the gymnasium where all the boys lined up on three sides of a square. For minor offences, a boy was laid face down across a long desk, feet strapped, while his shirt was pulled out over his head. Captain Hindrum, a retired Navy man, then gave him from three to six hefty strokes with a four-foot cane. Recipients would cry appallingly or even faint and afterwards have to be carried away to recover. For more serious offences, a birch was used: after three strokes, a boy needed to be taken to the surgery for treatment.[8]

District Schools, or 'barrack' schools as they were often disparagingly known, became the subject of much criticism. Not only were

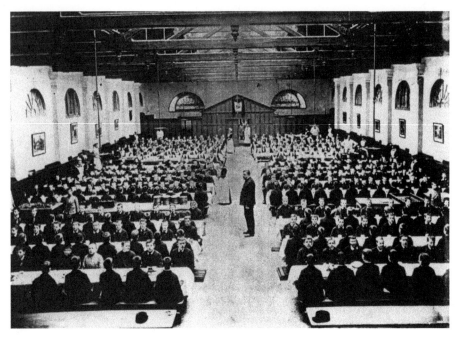

The dining hall of the Central London District Schools in Hanwell, also known as the Cuckoo Schools. Future film star Charlie Chaplin was an inmate of the Schools in the 1890s.

they expensive to operate, but also proved to be a breeding ground for infectious conditions such as ophthalmia (a serious eye complaint) and ringworm (a fungal condition for which Chaplin received treatment while at Hanwell – having his head shaved and stained brown with iodine). In the last quarter of the nineteenth century, alternative forms of children's accommodation were developed which were more flexible, economical and generally accepted as being better for the children who were placed there.

Certified Schools

In 1849, in the wake of the disastrous cholera outbreak at Mr Drouet's school, boards of guardians were forbidden to accommodate pauper children at privately run institutions. A relaxation on this stricture came in 1857 when guardians were permitted to board out children in Certified Industrial Schools (see chapter 2).

For groups wishing to 'rescue' children from what they viewed as the inappropriate surroundings of the workhouse, this provided the only mechanism available by which they could enter into a formal arrangement with a board of guardians for the purpose. To this end, a number of establishments subsequently applied for accreditation as Certified Industrial Schools, even though they had no desire to receive children placed by the courts under the 1857 Industrial Schools Act.

The matter was one of the subjects considered by the 1861 Parliamentary Select Committee on Poor Relief. One witness, Mrs Emmeline Way, described a girls' home she had opened two years earlier in Brockham, where orphaned or deserted girls were trained for domestic service. The establishment had originally been funded by charitable contributions. Since becoming a Certified Industrial School, however, Mrs Way had also received money both from the Privy Council, for girls committed by the courts, and from several boards of guardians, for workhouse girls they had sent to be trained as servants.

The Select Committee also heard representations from the Roman Catholic community alleging that workhouses often coerced Catholic children into participating in Anglican services and prayers.

As a result of the Committee's deliberations, the Poor Law (Certified Schools) Act of 1862 created a new class of institution known as the Certified School, which could receive children boarded out by guardians. The maximum rate of payment was based on what the cost of maintaining the child in the workhouse would have been. Parents of pauper children placed at a Certified School, who would almost certainly be in receipt of poor relief themselves, were not expected to contribute. As with Reformatory and Industrial Schools, Certified Schools were open to official inspection.

Several hundred Certified Schools were eventually in operation. As might be expected, they were particularly popular with the Roman Catholic community. In some cases, Catholic Certified Schools set their charging level well below the possible maximum in order to encourage guardians to take advantage of their accommodation. As well as saving money, the use of Certified Schools could also relieve guardians of the need to make special arrangements for the religious requirements of non-Anglican children in their care. Some Certified Schools specialized in the training of girls for domestic service – another task that the workhouse authorities were often happy to offload.

Cottage Homes

The use of children's cottage homes in England was pioneered by charitable establishments such as the Home for Little Boys founded

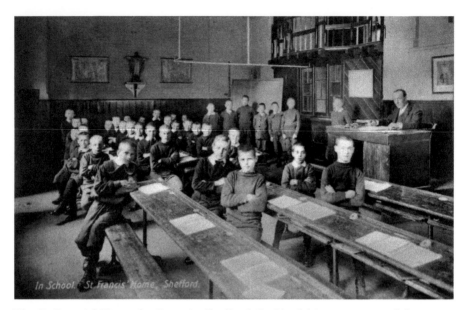

The St Francis' Home for Boys in Shefford, Bedfordshire, was one of the many Certified Schools established to receive Roman Catholic children.

in 1865 in Farningham, Kent, the Princess Mary's Homes for Little Girls established in 1870 in Addlestone, Surrey, and the Barnardo's Village Home for Girls in Barkingside, Essex, opened in 1876. In each case, the children were accommodated in a purpose-built 'village' of small houses set around a central green. In each house, a group of girls or boys of varying ages lived under the supervision of a house mother. As well as houses and a school, the facilities could include an infirmary, chapel, workshops, bakehouse and laundry. Boys were taught practical trades such as shoemaking, tailoring, plumbing and joinery, while girls learned household skills such as sewing, cooking and cleaning to equip them for domestic service.

Adoption of the cottage homes system for pauper children was proposed in an 1874 report to the Local Government Board by Mrs Jane Senior,[9] the first female Poor Law inspector. She was also daughter-in-law of the economist Nassau Senior, one of the architects of the New Poor Law. This close family connection did not however prevent her from becoming a fierce critic of the system, particularly in the way it dealt with children. She criticized the existing 'barrack' schools that had been set up by a number of Poor Law authorities as being breeding grounds for disease and also failing to give their inmates any individual attention. Cottage homes, housing children in household groups of 'no more than 20 to 30' in a rural environment, would, she said, be 'of a more home-like character' and provide a 'free and natural mode of life'.[10]

In the mid-1870s, the Poor Law unions of West Derby, West Ham and Bolton made tentative experiments with the cottage homes approach, although each used buildings erected on their existing workhouse sites. The West Derby and West Ham homes also housed fifty children – rather more than the maximum proposed by Mrs Senior. The first true Poor Law cottage home developments were established in South Wales by the unions in Swansea (1877), Neath (1878) and Bridgend and Cowbridge (1879), with schemes in England being opened by Birmingham (1879) and the Kensington and Chelsea School District (1880).

Like their voluntary counterparts, the larger Poor Law cottage homes sites sometimes included facilities such as a gymnasium or swimming bath, and often established a boys' military band which could provide a pathway into a career as a musician in the army or navy.

By the 1920s, around 115 Poor Law unions operated premises which they described as cottage homes although some barely deserved the description, consisting of just one or two houses located near the workhouse.

Isolated/Scattered Homes

The 'isolated homes' system was devised in 1893 by John Wycliffe Wilson, Chairman of the Sheffield Board of Guardians. Wycliffe Wilson criticized the by then well-established cottage homes system as isolating children from the real world in which they would eventually have to make their way. The alternative system of boarding out (see chapter 17), though well regarded, relied on a steady supply of foster families, which was not always guaranteed. It was also only appropriate for orphans and deserted children, and was also not suited for short-term inmates such as the 'ins and outs' – those who repeatedly entered and the workhouse and left after a short stay.

Isolated homes, or scattered homes as they became more commonly known, placed small groups of children in ordinary houses scattered around the suburbs of Sheffield. Unlike cottage home sites which usually had their own schools, the children in scattered homes attended ordinary local Board Schools. The placing of homes was arranged such that there were never more than thirty scattered homes children attending any one school.

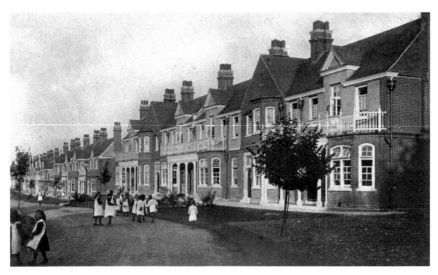

Girls at play at the Poplar Union Schools in Hutton, Essex, early 1900s. As well as the cottage homes, each housing 30 children, the site had its own schools, infirmary, chapel and swimming pool.

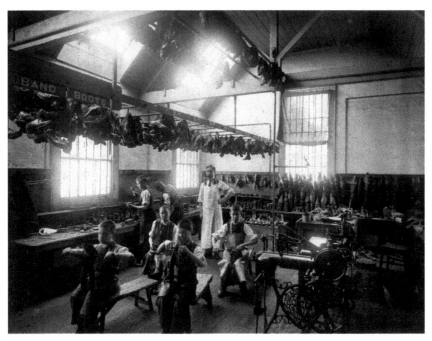

Boot- and shoe-making workshop at the Kensington & Chelsea School District cottage homes, early 1900s. Band boots hang from a rail above.

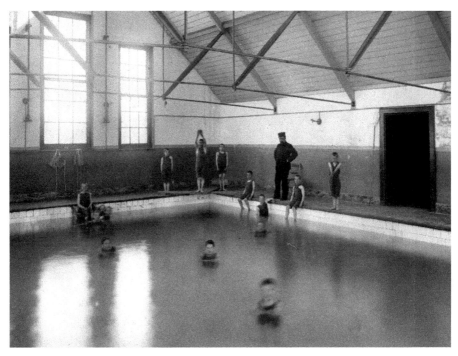

Swimming bath at the Kensington & Chelsea School District cottage homes site in Banstead, Surrey, early 1900s.

Initially, Sheffield had nine homes each containing between fifteen and twenty-eight beds. Seven of the homes were allocated to Protestant children and two to Roman Catholics. Each house was presided over by a foster mother, assisted in the household work by the elder children and an occasional charwoman.

Similar schemes were adopted by many other unions beginning with Whitechapel and Bath in 1897. In some cases, a union would take over or even erect a small row of ordinary houses in a normal residential area. In 1913, the West Ham union had around a dozen houses used as scattered homes including a block at 21–27 Pelham Road, South Woodford.

Unions which had a large number of scattered homes usually erected a headquarters home which acted as a receiving or probationary home for new arrivals, short-term inmates, and those requiring special supervision. The headquarters home also providing an administrative and supplies base for the outlying homes.

By 1914, over ninety unions were making use of scattered homes. Although some of the urban establishments run by voluntary

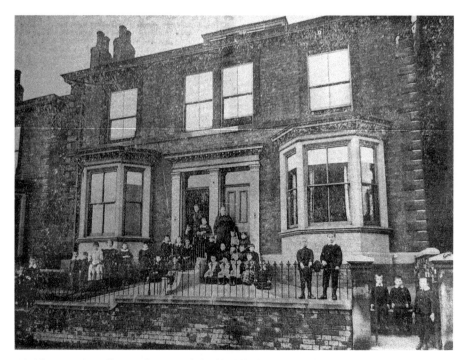

Children and staff outside one of Sheffield's first scattered homes in about 1898.

bodies were similar in character to scattered homes, use of the term is particularly associated with those run by the Poor Law authorities.

Training Ships

Training ships (see chapter 4) provided another option for removing boys from the workhouse, with the Local Government Board regularly promoting their use. Boards of guardians, however, appear to have shown some reluctance in taking advantage of the vessels – in 1911, the national total of Poor Law boys placed on the ten ships then available was only 453. This may have partly been due to the cost of maintaining them there, typically eight or nine shillings a week, which was generally a little higher than keeping them in a union's own accommodation. A payment might also be required for a boy's uniform.

A speaker at the 1904 Central Poor Law Conference extolled the virtues of training ships as a way of improving the prospects of boys from impoverished backgrounds. There was, he suggested, 'the substantial fact that a boy who goes from the *Exmouth* into a naval training ship can at the age of 40 secure a pension of over £50 for life.[11]

Pauper Emigration

Although the 1834 Poor Law Amendment provided for the parish-funded emigration of the poor, it was not until that late 1840s that emigration began to be targeted at pauper children.

In 1848, the Colonial Land and Emigration Commissioners (CLEC) launched a drive to encourage immigration to South Australia and New South Wales. It was proposed that orphans between the ages of 14 and 18, who were of industrious habits and good character, free from all disease, and having been vaccinated against smallpox, should be considered for emigration. They would also be required to have a sufficient knowledge of reading, writing and arithmetic, and the principles of the Christian religion. Orphanhood was defined as having lost at least one parent. Female orphans were much preferred as candidates for emigration because males greatly outnumbered females in these colonies.

The orphan emigration scheme was taken up by Ireland's PLC at a time when the Great Famine was just beginning to subside. The Irish Commissioners decided, however, to confine its use to females. In the first year of the operation, 2,219 girls emigrated from Irish workhouses with another 1,056 the following year.[12] The scheme was discontinued in 1850 after complaints that most of the girls arriving in Australia were of disreputable character and lacked training in domestic skills.

The emigration of the poor from mainland Britain was given a boost in the late 1840s by two changes in the law. First, under the Poor Law Amendment Act of 1848, the financing of emigration could be charged to a common fund within each union, rather than having to be funded by the parish in which an emigrant was settled. Second, the 1850 Poor Law Amendment Act provided that a union could undertake the emigration of any 'poor orphan or deserted child under the age of sixteen years' that was in its care. The resulting increase in emigration peaked at a total of 3,271 in 1852 and then, as in Ireland, declined to just a few hundred a year.

An End to Children in Workhouses

In 1913, the Local Government Board decreed that no healthy child over the age of 3 should be living in a workhouse after 1915. The intervention of the First World War slowed progress in achieving this goal, but at the start of 1922 just over 5 per cent of such children were in 'general' institutions, i.e. workhouses, although most of these were in special children's wards. At the same date, the overall total of 64,152 children in Poor Law institutions in England and Wales included 9,279 in scattered homes, 10,847 in cottage homes, 5,113 in District Schools, 6,181 in 'other homes' and 749 on training ships. An additional 9,782 children were being boarded out, with around 17 per cent living outside their home union. A total of 9,485 children were housed in establishments not run by Poor Law authorities, of which 6,134 were in institutions – largely privately run – licensed under the 1862 Certified Schools Act.[13] By 1922, there were 217 schools certified for this purpose, most described as 'small orphanages'.[14]

Chapter 16

Emigration Homes

As Thomas Barnardo's biographers were to put it, 'an ever-open entrance to the Homes demands an ever-open exit'.[1] For many of the organizations that operated children's homes, the continuing 'disposal' of a significant proportion of the existing inmates was always a concern if places were to remain available for new arrivals. The two most widely adopted solutions to this problem were boarding out (fostering), which will be discussed in the next chapter, and emigration.

Apart from freeing up institutional places for new arrivals, emigration had economic attractions. The one-off cost of a passage to Canada, typically in the order of £10, compared very favourably to the recurring cost of keeping a child in residential care which might amount to as much as £16 a year. By the end of the nineteenth century, child emigration was also seen as a patriotic endeavour with the young colonists forming 'the bricks with which the Empire would be built'.[2]

The emigration schemes operated by some of the larger charities have already been described. This chapter examines some of the other agencies involved in this activity and the homes that were established in Britain to prepare children for their impending emigration to countries such as Canada and Australia.

Interest in children's emigration rose rapidly from the late 1860s, largely due to the activities of two women, Miss Maria Rye and Miss Annie Macpherson, who independently began organizing the emigration and resettlement of children in Canada. Their numerous clients included the Poor Law authorities, the operators of Reformatory and Industrial Schools, and the growing number of charitable organizations that ran children's homes. The children emigrating from these various establishments have come to be known as British Home Children.

Maria Rye

Maria Rye was born in London in 1829, the daughter of a solicitor. In 1859, her growing concern over the lack of employment opportunities for young middle-class women led her to start up a law stationery business to provide work for such girls. She subsequently helped establish a Telegraph School to train women as telegraph clerks, and in 1861 co-founded the Female Middle-Class Emigration Society to help educated young women emigrate to the British colonies. After several years of escorting parties of women and girls to Australia, New Zealand and Canada, Miss Rye turned her attention to orphan and 'gutter' children, proposing their emigration to rural Canada and the western states of America. She took a group of three orphans to Canada in June 1869, followed in October of that year by a group of seventy-three children, aged from 4 to 17, including forty-nine from the Liverpool Board of Guardians' Industrial School in Kirkdale.[3]

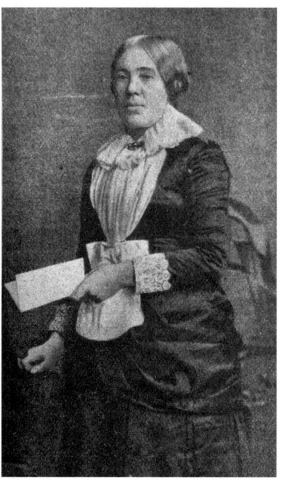

A portrait of Maria Rye (1829–1903), one of the leading promoters of children's emigration.

A large property known as Avenue House, on Peckham High Street in South London, became the base for the new enterprise. 'Miss Rye's Emigration Home for Destitute Little Girls' was opened in 1872, its object being 'to receive destitute little girls and send them to Canada, where they are placed out in families to be trained for service, the younger ones being adopted by patrons, and brought up as their own children'. Avenue House was run by Miss Rye's sister Elizabeth, or Bessie. Prior to their emigration, girls usually spent two or three months at the home receiving training in housework, kitchen work and laundry work, to equip them for future employment as domestic servants.

Miss Rye established a Canadian base in a former courthouse and gaol in Niagara-on-the-Lake in Ontario. The property, which she named Our Western Home, was adapted to act as a holding home for 120 children. In 1874, following adverse reports about the treatment received by some of the pauper children Miss Rye had placed in Canada, and suggestions she was personally profiting from public funds she had received, an inquiry was conducted by Local Government Board inspector Mr Andrew Doyle. Doyle visited Canada to interview around 400 children who had emigrated under Miss Rye's care and his report, published in 1875, expressed serious concerns relating to their welfare and aftercare. He found that young children tended to be adopted, and were generally well placed and treated with kindness and affection. Some older children were apprenticed or went into domestic service, but the majority were placed in farm service. Many who went into service suffered hardship, ill-treatment and deprivation. Many children had not been visited for several years and others had been lost track of altogether.[4]

Although Doyle's findings were vigorously disputed by Miss Rye, the emigration of pauper children was halted until 1883, mainly due to the lack of adequate ongoing superintendence of the children in their new homes. Despite this setback, Miss Rye continued her activities and over a twenty-five-year period placed around 5,000 girls in new homes in Canada.

When Miss Rye retired in 1895, she donated Avenue House to the Waifs and Strays Society, together with her Canadian reception home in Niagara-on-the-Lake. Avenue House, which no longer stands, then became the Society's Peckham Emigration Home.

Annie Macpherson

Annie Macpherson, a Scottish Evangelical Quaker, was four years junior to Miss Rye. She moved to London in 1865 where she took up

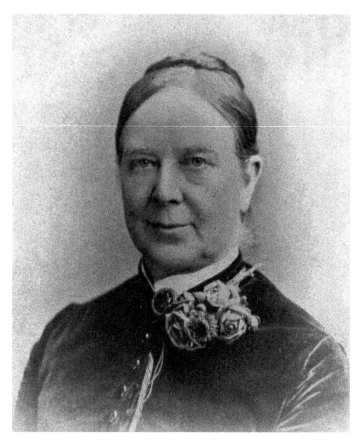

Annie Macpherson (1833–1904) was another leading figure in the child emigration movement, in which many of her family also became involved.

mission work among the young female matchbox makers in the East End. The following year, she turned to providing accommodation for destitute children and rented a house in Hackney as a home for thirty boys. It was known as a Revival Refuge as financial support for its opening had come from readers of the evangelical newspaper *The Revival*. A second home for a further thirty boys followed, located at the rear of Shoreditch church.

In 1868, she acquired premises at 60 Commercial Street, in the Spitalfields district. The building, originally a warehouse, had previously been used as a cholera hospital run by the Sisters of Mercy and was fitted throughout with gas and water supplies. The new home, named the 'Home of Industry', opened in February 1869 and provided food, shelter, work, basic education and religious instruction for up to 200 inmates.

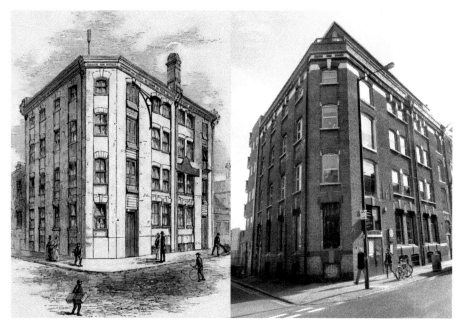

Opened in 1868, Miss Macpherson's House of Industry at 60 Commercial Street, Spitalfields, is now used as commercial premises.

Faced with the problem of the seemingly limitless numbers of children needing help, Miss Macpherson became an active promoter of child emigration. From 1870 onwards, she regularly took parties of children to Canada where she established reception homes in Belleville and Galt in Ontario, and Knowlton in Quebec, from where they were placed with new families. The children she migrated were drawn both from her own homes and also other agencies such as Barnardo's, the Quarrier's Homes in Scotland and the Smyly Homes in Dublin, as well as some from workhouses.

Miss Macpherson expanded her work back in England with the opening of a Training Farm in Hampton in Middlesex. A girls' home was also opened in Hampton but was found to be inconveniently far out of London for its staff to travel to and was closed in 1874. It was replaced by a new home in London Fields, Hackney. In 1887, the Home of Industry moved to purpose-built premises at 29 Bethnal Green Road, London.

Miss Macpherson retired in 1902 and died two years later at her retirement home in Hove. Her organization was taken over in 1920 by the Liverpool Sheltering Home.

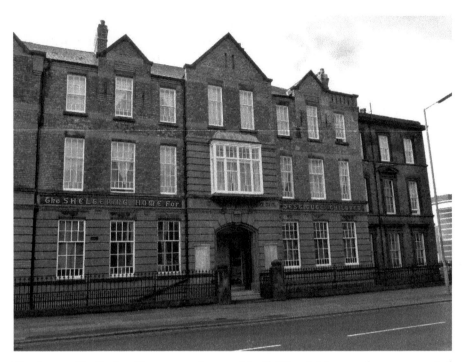

The former Sheltering Home premises on Myrtle Street, Liverpool, now occupied by the John Moores University.

Liverpool Sheltering Home

In 1872, Annie Macpherson was invited to give a talk about her work to a group of Liverpool shipowners who had become concerned at the numbers of destitute and orphaned children in the city. Due to other commitments, her place was taken by her sister, Mrs Louisa Birt, who had been assisting with her work in London. Birt was persuaded to stay in Liverpool to take charge of a new establishment, the Liverpool Sheltering Home, whose main role was to be the emigration of suitable children. A link was established with a wealthy farmer in Nova Scotia who initially organized accommodation for children emigrating from the Home. Then, from 1876, use was made of the reception home that Miss Macpherson had established in Knowlton.

In 1889, the Sheltering Home moved into purpose-built premises on Myrtle Street, Liverpool, where 120 children could be accommodated. According to an 1894 directory:

> *The object of the home is to afford to boys and girls who have lost father, mother or both parents, elementary education, scriptural*

instruction and a short industrial training, and then to provide homes or situations for them in Canada; girls are admitted between the ages of 4 and 16, and boys between 10 and 16, upon the approval of the superintendent, without votes or other interest, and the home is entirely undenominational; this institution is wholly supported by voluntary contributions: the cost of training, out fitting and emigrating a child is £10; already nearly 3,500 children have been emigrated after a very careful training in the home, and 95 per cent are found to have done well.[5]

Louisa Birt continued as superintendent of the Sheltering Home until her death in 1915 although she had ceased active work several years before. During her lifetime, around 6,000 children from the Homes had emigrated to Canada. In 1925, the establishment was taken over by Barnardo's who continued its operation although it now only took boys of working age due to changes in Canadian immigration regulations. It finally closed in 1935 and was sold to Liverpool Corporation for use as a Juvenile Employment Centre. The building is now occupied by part of Liverpool's John Moores University.

Middlemore Homes

In Birmingham, in 1872, John Throgmorton Middlemore, the son of a wealthy leather manufacturer, founded the Children's Emigration Homes. At first, the Homes occupied a number of separate premises in the city, but were eventually brought together in large premises on St Luke's Road, in the Highgate district. The Emigration Homes were entirely directed to giving children practical training in preparation for life and work in Canada – the girls were taught domestic skills, while the boys learned manual trades. Having made arrangements for their reception in Toronto, Middlemore set sail for Canada with his first party of twenty-six children on 1 May 1873 on board the SS *Sarmatian*. A further group of fifty children made the crossing in May 1874 aboard the SS *Prussian*. In 1875, a receiving home for Middlemore children, known as Guthrie House, was established in London, Ontario.

As well as children from his own homes, from 1887 onwards Middlemore also took children to Canada on behalf of other institutions such as the Wolverhampton, Chelsea, St Olave's and St George in the East Poor Law Unions, and the Shustoke Industrial School. Conversely, children from the Middlemore homes were sometimes taken across with other emigration organizers such as Miss Macpherson.

Middlemore continued his active involvement in the Homes until his death in October 1924. In recognition of his work, the Emigration Homes were renamed the Middlemore Homes in 1925.

From the mid-1920s, Canada became more restrictive in its policy towards child immigration and Australia gradually became the main destination for British Home Children, with many of those from the Middlemore Homes then starting their new lives at the Fairbridge Farm School in Western Australia.

In 1928, The Middlemore Homes moved to new purpose-built premises on Weoley Park Road, Selly Oak. A babies' home was added to the establishment in May 1939.

Following a steep decline in numbers immigrating to Australia after 1948, the Weoley Park Road property was leased to the Birmingham City Council who used it as a children's home known as Middlemore House. The home closed in 1955 and the site later became part of Westhill College, now demolished.

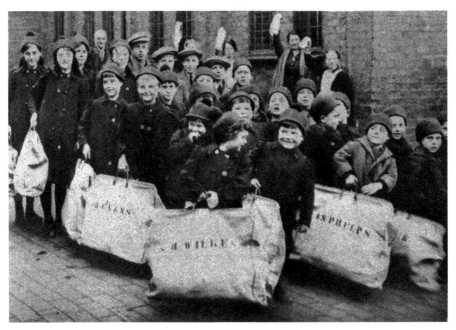

A party of children departing for Canada from the Middlemore Emigration Homes in 1920. Each carries a name-stencilled canvas bag containing their clothes and other possessions.

Other Emigration Homes

In around 1871, after meeting Annie Macpherson on a visit to Toronto, Mrs Margaret Blaikie returned home to Edinburgh and founded the Emigration Home, also known as the Canadian Home, on Lauriston Lane. Over the next twenty years, she organized the immigration to Canada of about 300 children.

The Manchester and Salford Boys' and Girls' Refuges established two emigration homes. A training home for girls, known as Rosen Hallas, was opened by the charity in 1886 at Cheetham Hill. A boys' emigration home was established in 1891 on Great Ducie Street, Manchester.

The large Barnardo homes at Barkingside and Stepney Causeways played an ongoing role in preparing children for emigration. A further facility was added in 1882 with the opening of the Labour House on Commercial Road in East London. It provided lodgings and work for up to 120 boys aged 17 or over, many of whom immigrated to Canada, initially being received at Barnardo's Industrial Farm near Russell, Manitoba. The Labour House eventually closed in 1909.

The Waifs and Strays Society had several homes which were particularly involved in the preparation of boys for emigration. The

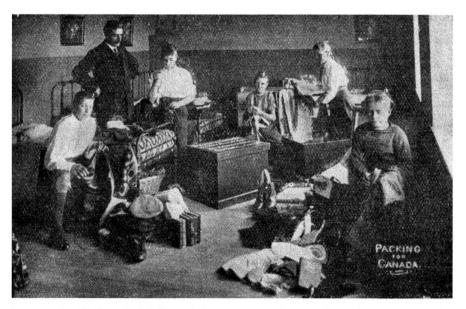

Boys at the St Benet's Waifs and Strays Society home, Caversham, packing for Canada.

earliest was the Boys' Farm Home opened in 1885 at Standon Bridge in Staffordshire. It was followed by Hedgerley Court Farm Home for Boys, in Buckinghamshire, established in 1893, and St Benet's Gardening Home for Boys opened in 1903 in Caversham. A home for girls was added in 1895 following Miss Rye's gift to the Society of Avenue House in Peckham.

In 1911, James Fegan had the idea of setting up a 'Canada Training Farm' to prepare boys prior to their emigration for the kind of work they were most likely to end up doing in their new country. On hearing about the scheme, a City merchant met with Fegan and commissioned him to buy fifty acres of suitable land with the promise of £3,000 to start the venture. The site he selected for the 'farm colony' was in Great Hordern, near Goudhurst, in Kent. Within a few months of its purchase, fifty boys had been installed, farm implements ordered from Canada, and the building of extensive premises begun.

The use of emigration by Reformatory and Industrial Schools was rather variable as its cost could not be covered by the official allowances they received for the maintenance of their inmates. Institutions that had the benefit of income from other sources, such as charitable donations, were much better able to employ emigration for the disposal of those in their charge. One such establishment was the Redhill Farm School for Boys, run by the Philanthropic Society – a notable advocate of emigration. Up to the end of 1881, a total of 2,891 boys had passed through the Reformatory's doors, of whom almost half (1,302) had been migrated at their time of discharge.[6]

Chapter 17

Boarding Out/Fostering

Boarding out – now more usually known as fostering – became widely used for placing destitute or orphan children, often for a long period, in the care of foster parents who usually received a weekly allowance for each child staying with them. The system is said to have originated in Scotland, where it was in operation from at least the sixteenth century.[1] Its use was officially sanctioned in England and Wales by Gilbert's Act of 1782 which provided that 'all Infant Children of tender Years, and who, from Accident or Misfortune, shall become chargeable to the Parish or Place to which they belong, may ... be placed ... with some reputable Person or Persons in or near the Parish, Township, or Place, to which they belong, at such weekly Allowance as shall be agreed upon between the Parish Officers and such Person or Persons'.[2]

The development of boarding out in the Victorian era owed much to its take-up by the Poor Law authorities. Much of its attraction was due to financial considerations, in that it could prove more economical and flexible than providing institutional accommodation. Boarding out first came under official consideration by the central Poor Law authority, the Poor Law Board, in 1868. Up until then, the Board had been informally opposed to the system since it handed over the control of children to those whose main aim might simply be to make a profit from the weekly maintenance payments they received. Fears of possible neglect, cruelty or exploitation of boarded out children made the Board extremely cautious about sanctioning its use. In 1869, the Board asked its inspectors to report on the use of boarding out in England and Wales. It was discovered that twenty-one Poor Law unions in England and Wales were using boarding out, covering a total of 347 children, generally with good results. One union, Warminster, had successfully used boarding out for more than twenty years. The Board also commissioned a report from one of their inspectors, Mr Henley, on the operation of boarding out in Scotland. Henley noted some particular attributes of the Scots – their generally good level of education, and the existence of a class of crofters or small occupiers (a class relatively unknown in England) who proved to be good foster parents.[3]

The Poor Law Board agreed to a wider trial of boarding out and in 1870 issued a formal framework for its use. The Boarding-out Order specified that:

- A Boarding-out Committee be formed in each union to supervise the boarding-out arrangements – Committees were to have at least three members at least one of which was to be female.
- Only orphans and deserted children to be boarded out.
- Only children aged between two and ten to be boarded out.
- No more than two children to be boarded out in the same home unless brothers and sisters.
- No child to be boarded out with foster parents of a different religious persuasion.
- Foster parents to sign an undertaking agreeing to 'bring up the child as one of their own children, and provide it with proper food, lodging, and washing, and endeavour to train it in habits of truthfulness, obedience, personal cleanliness, and industry, as well as suitable domestic and outdoor work'.
- Weekly maintenance fee not to exceed four shillings a week.
- No child to be boarded out in a home more than a mile-and-a-half from a suitable school
- No child to be boarded out in a home more than five miles from the residence of a Boarding-out Committee member.[4]

A revised order in 1877 prohibited the boarding out of children with foster parents who were themselves in receipt of poor relief. Further orders were issued in 1889 which also provided for the boarding out of children outside their own union. In 1885, the Local Government Board appointed a woman inspector, Miss Marianne Mason, who along with two female colleagues regularly visited the thousand or so children who were being boarded out beyond their own union.

By the end of the nineteenth century, around half of the unions in England and Wales were using boarding out, with around 8,000 orphaned or deserted children placed in homes. Although occasional cases of ill-treatment emerged, these were far outweighed by stories of children filled with dread at the possibility of being taken away from their foster homes. Although boarding out established itself as one of the most popular ways of dealing with children in the care of a union, it rarely proved possible to find enough families willing to take on the role. It was also only suitable for children in long-term care – for the many children who came and went more quickly, scattered homes were a more suitable solution.

After some initial caution, the use of boarding out was gradually taken up by the voluntary sector. Apart from offering an economical and flexible way of expanding the supply of accommodation, boarding out came to be regarded as the nearest approximation to a 'normal' home life that could be provided by a child care agency.

In 1887, Thomas Barnardo placed 330 boys aged from 5 to 9 with families in rural districts. The foster parents, who received 5/- a week for each child, had to sign a lengthy and detailed agreement as to how the children were to be treated. Regular inspection of the children was originally carried out by a specially employed female physician, with nurses later taking on the role.

In 1896, Barnardo's was boarding out more children than all the English Poor Law unions put together, even though the total number of children in the charge of these authorities was more than ten times as many as the children in the care of his organization.[5] One of the few complaints about the system was that when reaching the age of 14,

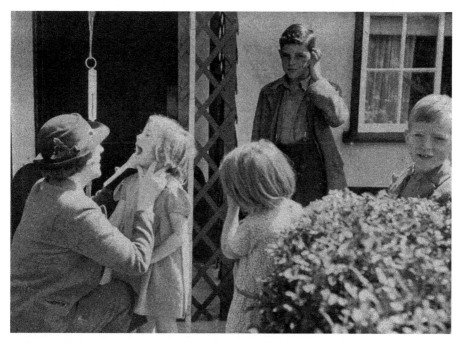

A Barnardo's inspector examines the mouth of a child being boarded out, late 1930s

children had to move back to one of the central homes to receive technical or domestic training – even though this might be after many years of living with the same foster family.

The Waifs and Strays Society made use of boarding out right from the start, with around a quarter of the children in the Society's care being fostered each year.[6] Much of the groundwork in finding foster homes was placed in the hands of local clergy who, together with other suitable people from the area, also supervised the children and submitted reports on them every three months. Regulations for fostering were instigated, based on those used by the Poor Law unions. The Society's version specified that children should normally not be boarded out above the age of 7, and never above ten. Boarding out was not to take place with relatives or anyone in receipt of poor relief. Payment was never to exceed five shillings a week.[7]

When receiving a child, foster parents entered into a formal contract with the organization placing it, such as the one shown on the following page made in 1908 between the Sheffield Poor Law Union and Isabella Crosby of Cockermouth in Cumberland. This also illustrates the long distance that children sometimes travelled to their foster home placements.

Despite supervision and regulations, cases of neglect or cruelty occasionally surfaced. In 1893, the Waifs and Strays Society appointed a professional inspectress who toured the country making unannounced visits to the Society's homes.

After a slow start, the National Children's Home (NCH) also made use of boarding out. In 1909, of the 7,924 children received by the charity, 2,008 were still in its care, of whom 477 (almost 24 per cent) were in foster homes.[8] In line with other agencies, the NCH brought fostered children back into one of its homes before they left its care. The age at which the NCH did this – 7 or 8 – was much lower than that applied in other organizations.

Boarding out came to the fore in 1946 following its endorsement by the Curtis Report as the preferred solution for children in care, unless adoption was a possibility. This conclusion was reinforced by the 1948 Children Act, which gave local councils a much greater role in the provision of welfare services for children (see chapter 20). It was also a development that was to present a serious challenge to many of the voluntary agencies. Although some of these organizations had previously made use of boarding out, the majority came from a deeply rooted tradition with the provision of institutional accommodation at its heart. The new emphasis on fostering was a

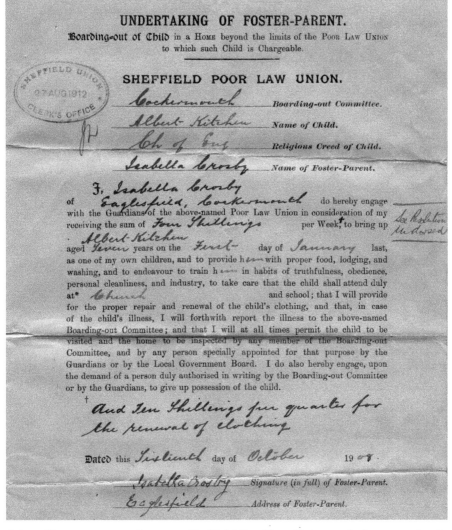

UNDERTAKING OF FOSTER-PARENT.

Boarding-out of Child in a Home beyond the limits of the Poor Law Union to which such Child is Chargeable.

SHEFFIELD POOR LAW UNION.

Cockermouth ———— *Boarding-out Committee.*

Albert Kitchen ———— *Name of Child.*

Ch of Eng ———— *Religious Creed of Child.*

Isabella Crosby ———— *Name of Foster-Parent.*

I, *Isabella Crosby* of *Eaglesfield, Cockermouth* do hereby engage with the Guardians of the above-named Poor Law Union in consideration of my receiving the sum of *Four Shillings* per Week, to bring up *Albert Kitchen* aged *Seven* years on the *First* day of *January* last, as one of my own children, and to provide her with proper food, lodging, and washing, and to endeavour to train her in habits of truthfulness, obedience, personal cleanliness, and industry, to take care that the child shall attend duly at* *Church* and school; that I will provide for the proper repair and renewal of the child's clothing, and that, in case of the child's illness, I will forthwith report the illness to the above-named Boarding-out Committee; and that I will at all times permit the child to be visited and the home to be inspected by any member of the Boarding-out Committee, and by any person specially appointed for that purpose by the Guardians or by the Local Government Board. I do also hereby engage, upon the demand of a person duly authorised in writing by the Boarding-out Committee or by the Guardians, to give up possession of the child.

And Ten Shillings per quarter for the renewal of clothing

Dated this *Sixteenth* day of *October* 19 *08* .

Isabella Crosby ———— *Signature (in full) of Foster-Parent.*

Eaglesfield ———— *Address of Foster-Parent.*

A boarding-out contract between Sheffield Poor Law Union and a foster mother in Cockermouth, Cumberland, for the care of seven-year-old Albert Kitchen. Long-distance placements were not uncommon.

development that would have enormous consequences over the following decades.

It is probably fair to say that of all the various forms of residential care established by child care agencies, boarding out became the one that proved the most durable and it continues to play a central role to the present day.

Chapter 18

Aftercare and Preventive Work

For young people leaving the protection of a child care organization, typically at around the age of 15, the move to independent adult life could be difficult. Those in this situation had often spent many years in an institutional environment where daily life was strictly regulated and timetabled. To help such individuals, efforts were often made to help ease their transition to living in the outside world.

Many institutions organized employment for their leavers. For girls, this was most often in domestic service. In the case of the boys, the possibilities could be more varied, depending on the demands for workers in the local area. Occasionally, institutions would form ongoing arrangements for placing their former inmates. In some cases, as occasionally happened with Industrial Schools, this might follow on from local outside work that boys had undertaken while still inmates of the School. Employment arrangements could also be rather further afield. In the early 1900s, for example, some of the boys leaving the Industrial Schools in Leeds and Desford went to work on farms in Wales, while Liverpool's Roman Catholic Female Orphanage found good situations for many of its girls in France.[1]

Auxiliary Homes and Working Boys'/Girls' Homes

For those moving on from their care, some organizations operated an intermediate form of accommodation variously known as Auxiliary Homes or Homes for Working Boys (or Girls).

The term Auxiliary Home was most commonly used for premises established for this purpose by Reformatory and Industrial Schools. Like their parent institutions, the Homes were required to be officially inspected and certified for operation. Auxiliary Homes were usually located in urban areas and provided supervised hostel-style accommodation for anything up to a hundred inmates, though most were much smaller than this, typically having between ten and twenty places. As well as their halfway-house function, the Homes often provided short-term accommodation for former inmates who were between situations or who were simply paying a social visit back to the institution.

More broadly speaking, the term Auxiliary Home could be applied to any annexe of a larger establishment, whatever its use. Other uses of Auxiliary Homes included the provision of overflow accommodation for ordinary inmates, and short-term occupation for holiday or convalescent purposes.

Homes for Working Boys/Girls fulfilled a similar role to Auxiliary Homes in providing supported hostel accommodation for young people entering the labour market. Some Working Homes were established as offshoots of the larger establishments run by various child care organizations. Others were operated by bodies which specifically focused on the working young. The latter group included organizations such as Homes for Working Boys in London, founded in 1870 to support 'boys between 13 and 17 years of age, who are in situations and earning wages, but who have no homes'.[2] A separate body, Homes for Working Girls in London, was set up in 1878 'to provide a home for those girls and young women, 15 to 25 years of age, working in factories and workrooms, or as milliners, who are homeless; to afford them profitable recreation and "to surround them with healthful influences and friendly guidance"'.[3] Other groups included the Metropolitan Association for Befriending Young Servants (MABYS), the London East End Hostel Association and the Manchester and Salford Refuges. In the 1950s and 1960s, as part of their increasing involvement in the welfare of children and young people, local councils in cities such as Birmingham, Bristol and Leicester, also set up hostels for those in the early stages of employment.

Monitoring Former Inmates

Many organizations tried to keep in touch with former inmates after they moved on. In some cases, girls entering domestic service were given encouragement to hold down their jobs by an award system. In the 1890s, girls leaving the Stafford County Industrial Home who retained their situation for at least a year, and received a good report from their employer, received a gratuity of one guinea and an outfit. Due to numbers of girls quitting their posts immediately after receiving this payment, the scheme was amended to spread the payment of the award over two years.

The aftercare responsibilities of the Poor Law authorities were laid down in the 1851 Poor Law (Apprentices) Act, which required each union's Relieving Officers to visit, at least twice a year, any person below the age of 16 who had been taken from the workhouse as a servant or apprentice. Any deficiencies in the treatment of such young persons were to be communicated to the board of guardians. However, the obligation for such supervision lasted only until the individuals reached the age of 16 or left their situation. The Poor Law Act of 1899 required that any child who was in a union's care and then adopted, was to be visited twice a year for a period of three years from the date of the adoption. During that period, the union's consent to the adoption could be revoked.

Metropolitan Association for Befriending Young Servants (MABYS)

A national scheme for the aftercare of pauper girls leaving the workhouse, especially those aged 16 or more, was suggested by the Poor Law inspector, Jane Senior. She had originally hoped that her proposal would be supported and funded by the state, but after it became clear that this would not be the case, she and her supporters – notably Henrietta Barnett – began a campaign to raise funds to establish a voluntary body. The new organization, known as the Metropolitan Association for Befriending Young Servants (MABYS), began work in 1875, with its activities confined to just the London area. By the 1890s, the Association had more than a thousand volunteers who visited girls at their workplaces, and helped them find accommodation and new employment, until they reached the age of twenty. MABYS and similar charitable organizations were helped by the 1879 Poor Law Act which allowed Boards of Guardians to contribute to their funds.

From 1882, the Local Government Board included a report from MABYS in its own annual report. During 1893, the Association had under its supervision 2,412 girls from London Poor Law Schools and 955 from other institutions. Of the total, 1,700 were reported as 'satisfactory in their conduct and work', 740 as 'those against whom no serious faults have been alleged', 189 as 'accused of dishonesty, untruth, extreme violence of temper etc.', and thirty-two as 'having lost character or been in prison for theft etc.'[4]

MABYS set up a number of its own establishments including a number of supervised hostels or lodging houses where girls could stay while looking for employment, free registry offices, where potential employers could place details of situations available and a training school. In the early 1900s, a number of MABYS establishments were certified as Auxiliary Homes, enabling them to receive girls who were leaving, or on licence from, Industrial Schools.

After the First World War, MABYS was renamed the Mabys Association for the Care of Young Girls. In 1943 its activities were taken over by the London County Council.

The Association for Befriending Boys was formed in 1898 and performed similar activities to MABYS within the London metropolitan area.

The Girls' Friendly Society (GFS)

The same year that MABYS was founded, 1875, also saw the launch of the Girls' Friendly Society (GFS), which aimed to provide friendship and support for the growing numbers of working-class country girls who were leaving home to take up employment in towns and cities.

The initiative for founding the GFS came from Mary Elizabeth Townsend, an Irish clergyman's daughter and wife of the artist Frederick Townsend. After Frederick inherited Honington Hall, his uncle's estate in Warwickshire, the couple became involved in local philanthropic activities. Mary helped in the work of the local girls' orphanage and became aware of the problems faced by girls going into domestic service, including loss of contact with their families and unwanted pregnancies which resulted in dismissal. After assisting in some diocesan 'rescue work' among 'fallen women', she came to the conclusion that prevention would be much better than cure.

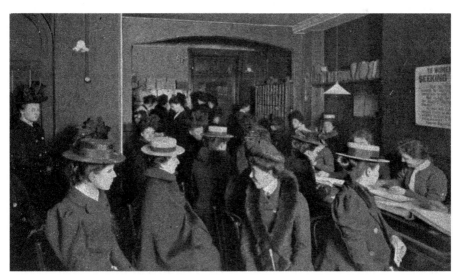

A London servants' registry, where those looking for a situation could be matched up with prospective employers.

The idea at the heart of the GFS was that the working-class girls who would form the Society's members would be befriended and guided by higher-class 'lady' associates. Girls could join the GFS from the age of 12, but from 1882 those from the age of 8 could become candidates, in preparation for membership. The Society operated within the parish and diocesan framework of the Church of England, with no branch being started without the consent of the local parish priest. All members were required to belong to the Church and be of unblemished character. Both members and associates paid an annual subscription.

GFS branches organized a variety of facilities for the Society's members. Girls seeking new situations could give their details to a GFS registry which could be consulted by prospective employers. Social activities were provided in comfortably furnished recreation rooms, supplied with newspapers, magazines, books and games. Hostels, known as Lodges, were set up in some towns and cities, including London, to provide cheaply priced food and lodgings. Accommodation was also set up for members who were domestic servants between situations. For girls 'toiling in close workrooms, and sometimes breaking down under the heavy strain of their task', Homes of Rest were established to provide rest, a change of air and scene, and a little motherly care, before resuming their employment.

Despite the broad similarity of their aims, there was no co-operation or co-ordination of effort between the GFS and MABYS, the two organizations holding rather different attitudes about whom they were prepared to assist. A GFS member had to be vouched for as being 'chaste' by a member of a class above her. The GFS also segregated former workhouse girls from its other members.[5] The Church of England affiliation of the GFS proved a barrier to Mrs Senior, and the non-sectarian, secular basis of the MABYS proved an anathema to Mrs Townsend. As Jane Senior's biographer put it, 'The GFS only wanted to help Anglican virgins; MABYS hoped to help non-Anglicans and non-virgins as well.'[6]

By 1880, the GFS had almost 40,000 members and over 13,500 associates. In the same year, Queen Victoria became the Society's Patron. In 1900, the Society had 1,361 branches with the members now numbering more than 150,000 and the associates almost 33,000. Branches also sprang up in many other countries.[7]

The advent of the First World War led to a drop in membership of the Society which then expanded its activities in many other directions. In 1921, the GFS took over a property in New Cross, known as Argyle House, which became a hostel for homeless girls and women and those escaping domestic violence. There was an increased focus on educational and training activities, cultural and sporting pursuits, and support for foreign travel.

During the Second World War, the GFS raised money for clubs and hostels for women working on the Home Front, while branches undertook various tasks from helping with evacuees to 'adopting' a minesweeper. In 1942, the Society launched a War Training Scheme for girls aged 14 to 18, which covered subjects ranging from Air Raid Precaution techniques to poultry keeping. A Youth Wartime Section provided housecraft training for girls aged 16 to eighteen.

In 1964, the Society began a development scheme to extend its work at home and abroad. New residential hostels for girls were opened in the large cities, most of which provided self-catering accommodation. The Society launched 'Girls at Work' courses in subjects such as fashion, make-up and etiquette, budgeting and interview techniques. There was also a scheme to operate lunch clubs for young working women.

The GFS is still active today, though no longer runs residential accommodation.

Ladies' Association for the Care of Friendless Girls

One of the most prominent organizations involved in 'preventive' work was the Ladies' Association for the Care of Friendless Girls (LA). The LA was founded in 1883 under the auspices of the Church of England, at the initiative of the women's campaigner Ellice Hopkins. The LA's focus was 'to prevent the degradation of women and children', in other words to prevent girls and women from falling into prostitution because of their social, economic or family or other circumstances. The LA operated as a confederation of locally run associations, which by 1885 numbered 106.

The LA had four main strands to its work. The Moral Education Branch sought to provide good moral teaching and to promote purity and chastity. This was aimed at both men and women, but still viewed women as being largely responsible for putting this into practice, with an emphasis on women's roles as wives and mothers.

The second strand, the Petitioning Branch, lobbied Parliament to take a stronger stand against prostitution, for example, by protecting girls from those who wished to seduce them. The Association's support was instrumental in the passing of the Criminal Law Amendment Act of 1885 which raised the age of female sexual consent from 13 to sixteen.

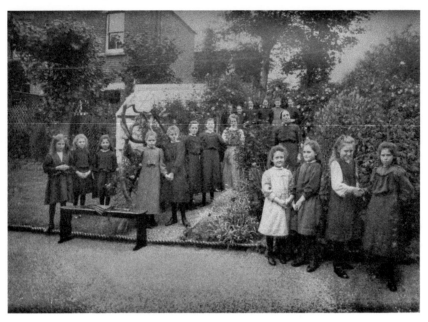

The matron and inmates of the Mount Hermon Home for Girls, Hastings, run by a branch of the Ladies' Association for the Care of Friendless Girls.

The Preventive Branch established training homes, registry offices and clothing clubs for domestic servants. The homes provided training in the skills of domestic service for girls considered at moral risk, with the registry helping trained girls to obtain a position or to move to a new one. Clothing clubs helped provide the uniform which girls were usually expected to possess when entering a new situation.

Finally, the Workhouse Magdalen Branch helped young, single, first-time mothers who, without family or other support, were often forced to enter workhouses. Such girls were viewed as particularly susceptible to resorting to prostitution in order to support themselves and their infant, the alternative being to give up the baby. The Associations tried to help girls find positions with a sympathetic employer and arrange fostering for the child. Some LA-run homes, such as those in Oxford, Exeter and Liverpool, eventually also provided accommodation for babies while their mothers worked elsewhere.

Ladies' Associations had largely disappeared by the Second World War. In some cases, the running of their residential homes – often given names such as the 'House of Help' – had been taken over by the local Anglican diocese or some other body.

Chapter 19

Magdalen Homes

Girls and women who had 'fallen', especially unmarried mothers or mothers-to-be, often became outcasts because of the shame that they brought on their families. Despite the circumstances that led many unfortunate young women into pregnancy, such as seduction under the promise of marriage, little distinction was made in the eyes of many between single mothers and prostitutes. In the latter part of the nineteenth century, the rescue and reform of young women in either situation became a major concern of charitable and religious groups, with a large number of establishments – generically referred to as Magdalen (or Magdalene) Homes – being set up to accommodate them. The Homes typically restricted admission to those up to the age of 25, with the lower age limit in some cases being as young as twelve. Where a pregnancy was involved, Homes would invariably only deal with 'first fall' cases, with 'repeat offenders' viewed as being beyond redemption.

In addition to the previously mentioned Salvation Army, Church Army and Ladies' Association, organizations operating Magdalen Homes included the Church Penitentiary Association, the Female Aid Society, the Roman Catholic Church and many independent local charities. Some offered temporary accommodation, usually free, while others required a stay of one or two years, with a weekly fee payable and work demanded. The aim of the long-stay homes, also known as Penitentiaries or Houses of Mercy, was the moral reform of their penitent inmates. The short-term establishments, sometimes referred to as Houses of Refuge, offered emergency shelter and could also act as probationary accommodation prior to entry into a Penitentiary.

The Penitentiary Regime

Life in Penitentiaries was strictly regulated and based on the belief that inmates, if they were to be reformed, required order in their lives and a strict regime of 'mild, wholesome, paternal, and Christian discipline'.[1] Daily life was characterized by a repetitive routine, the wearing of a uniform, plain food, work, religious instruction and attendance at services. Silence was often required for at least part of the day and especially in the dormitories. Freedom was usually restricted, with inmates barred from visiting friends or shops, or other influences that might tempt them away. All letters to or from inmates needed to be read by the matron before being passed on to the recipient. In some homes, those admitted were required to adopt a new name to reinforce their break with the past. At one Norwich institution, mothers or other female relatives could only visit inmates on the first Saturday of the month between 9 a.m. and 12 midday.[2] Privacy was often virtually non-existent. Inmates usually slept in dormitories and many institutions lacked private washing facilities. Here are the rules for the inmates at a typical late nineteenth-century home:

- Every girl is expected to rise when the bell rings, and to strip and shake up her bed, preparatory to making it when it is well aired.
- No talking is allowed in the bedrooms or lavatory or in the passages. Talking is allowed at meal times, after the girls have finished their meal.
- Silence is definitely expected from helpers and girls three times a day, viz.: 9 to 10 a.m., 2 to 3 p.m., 6.30 to 7.30 p.m.
- No grumbling is allowed except to the Superintendent herself, as no one else has power to remedy causes of grievance.
- No bad language is, of course, for one moment permitted, and no reference to girls' previous history allowed.
- No girl is permitted to make presents to anyone in the house, however trivial the gift may be.
- Every girl is expected to be obedient and respectful to all in authority.
- The girls are allowed to write letters once a month.[3]

All the household work such as scrubbing floors, making beds, preparing and cooking food, making and mending clothes, and washing uniforms and linen, was carried out by the inmates. Magdalen laundries have become particularly associated with Ireland, but they existed all across the British Isles. As well as dealing with the home's own laundry, washing was usually taken in from households in the locality. Apart from its practical use in providing work for the inmates and a valuable income for the institution, laundry work was also seen as having a symbolic dimension, signifying cleansing and purification.

Although institutions commonly required penitents to agree to remain for a minimum period, there were many instances of inmates making a premature departure, either with permission or by running away. In the latter case, the absconders could be taken to court for the theft of their uniform. Homes occasionally resorted to more extreme measures. In 1876, the Manchester and Salford Asylum resorted to adding several feet to the height of its walls to prevent inmates escaping.[4]

Domestic service was the eventual destination of some Magdalen inmates, though often with out-of-town employers, where a girl's history could be put behind her. Others ended up in low-grade and low-paid employment, such as laundry work. Some returned to their families and effectively became unpaid servants.

One of the earliest Magdalen institutions was the Magdalen Hospital for the Reception of Penitent Prostitutes, established in 1758 at 21 Prescot Street, Whitechapel – then a very insalubrious location with many brothels and drinking houses. Despite its name, the Hospital was not a medical facility. It received girls and women, below the age of 30, who had entered into prostitution but wished to reform, especially those who had not long 'fallen'. The inmates of the institution were occupied in laundry work and needlework and given religious instruction. The institution had a long life, eventually becoming an Approved School prior to its eventual closure in the 1960s.

An analysis[5] of Magdalen Hospital inmates from the institution's opening in 1758 until 1916 gives an overview of their eventual fate:

Placed in service or returned to friends	9,261
Lunatics or incurables	126
Died	135
Discharged at their own request	3,132
Discharged for improper conduct	1,473
In the Home, January, 1916	108
Total admissions	14,235

Around two-thirds of those admitted had what the Hospital would view as a successful outcome. The figure for those 'discharged at their own request' may well conceal a number who simply ran away from the establishment.

A notable provincial Magdalen Home was the House of Mercy in Horbury, near Wakefield, run by the Anglican Sisterhood of St Peter the Apostle. Its object was 'reclaiming fallen women and training them in the pursuit and practice of industry, virtue and Christian principles'. It opened in 1859, in a small cottage, accommodating around a dozen girls. Burgeoning demand for places led to plans being made for purpose-built

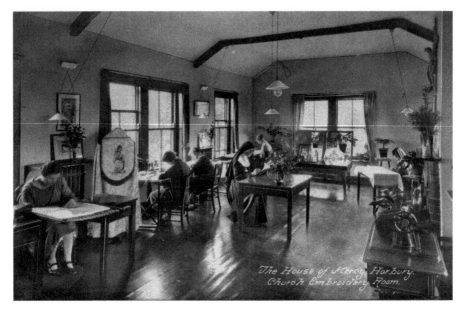

Inmates of the House of Mercy, Horbury, at work in the Church Embroidery Room.

permanent premises with space for up to eighty girls. The new building, whose construction cost £5,000, was opened in 1865. A certificate of good health was required for new entrants, who were expected to remain for two years. A £5 entrance fee or a weekly payment was requested when possible. Training was given in laundry work, needlework, embroidery, crochet work and dress-making. In 1943, Horbury was certified to operate as an Approved School for up to sixty senior girls who, like the home's voluntary inmates, were given training in domestic and laundry work, and also instructed in gardening.

Penitentiary Organizations

The Church Penitentiary Association (CPA), which was affiliated with the Church of England, was founded in 1852 'for the reformation of fallen women who have been servants or others'. By 1889, the Association's member institutions included 40 Penitentiaries, with accommodation for 1,250, and 36 Houses of Refuge, with accommodation for 247 penitents.[6]

A typical CPA member was the Kent Penitentiary, founded in 1860, and from 1866 located in Stone, near Dartford, where it adopted the name St Mary's. The home received admissions sent by clergymen, district visitors, and sometimes brought by their own friends. Girls applying at the door were treated with caution – they might be in hiding from the police or looking for free lodgings for a few days. New arrivals spent several months as probationers in a separate section of the building. They then moved to working in the laundry department until a vacancy came about in one of the 'house' departments.[7] The daily routine at the home began with a silent breakfast at 7 a.m., although a few girls rose at 6 to light fires and prepare breakfast. Following chapel at 7.30, work commenced at eight o'clock. At 11, the 'house girls' took up needlework. Dinner-time for all was at 12.30, followed by a ten-minute service in the chapel at one. The girls could then amuse themselves in the garden or classrooms until two, at which time they returned to their work which continued until 7.30 p.m. apart from a break for tea at five o'clock. After an hour spent in recreation, Bible class or chapel service, came supper at 8.30, prayers at nine o'clock, and bed at 9.30.[8]

Another important body was the Reformatory and Refuge Union set up in 1856 by the evangelical wing of the Church of England. The Union acted as an umbrella body for a wide range of groups involved in preventive, rescue and reform work. Its 1912 directory catalogued a total of 370 Magdalen institutions operating in England and Wales, of which 113 were in London. Between them, they provided almost 8,000 places.[9]

A major contribution in the capital was made by the London Female Preventive and Reformatory Institution (LFPRI). The organization was founded in 1857 'to seek the destitute and fallen by voluntary missionary effort; to afford temporary protection to friendless young women whose circumstances expose them to danger; to rescue fallen females, especially those decoyed from the country; to restore, when practicable, the wanderer to her family and friends, whether in town or country'.[10] It eventually operated around a dozen Magdalen Homes in the London area. Inmates were typically employed in housework, needlework, washing and other tasks up until 7 p.m., at the discretion of the home's matron. Time was also allowed for self-improvement, such as writing and reading. In the 1920s, LFPRI took over the work of another rescue organization, the Midnight Meeting Movement for the Rescue and Reclamation of Fallen Women, founded in 1859. By 1939, LFPRI's aims were stated as being 'to train destitute friendless girls for domestic service; to shelter virtuous young women in circumstances of moral peril; to seek and reclaim the betrayed and outcast'.[11] Reconciliations were also effected with relatives. After the Second World War, LFPRI became the London Haven for Women and Girls. Due to financial problems, the organization was finally wound up in 1976.

Changing Times

For a long period, Magdalen Homes made little or no provision for the accommodation of babies. New mothers were expected to have arranged for their infants to be looked after by relatives or friends, boarded out or given up for private adoption. By the start of the twentieth century, this was slowly changing, with a growing number of institutions starting to provide mother and baby places, some even incorporating the term into their name, such as the Cornwall Preventive and Rescue Association Mothers' and Babies' Home, founded in 1917, in St Agnes. The St Joseph's Home for Mothers and Babies, opened in Stockwell in 1922, was advertised as being for 'Roman Catholic unmarried expectant mothers and mothers with their babies on leaving hospital, first cases only'.[12]

In Britain, by the Second World War, the term 'Magdalen Home' was falling out of use although many of the institutions previously referred to by that name were still in operation, often rebranded as Training Homes. This was the case with the establishment in Horbury, which in 1946 was renamed St Peter's Training School.

During the 1960s, the increasing availability of the contraceptive pill, coupled with changes in social attitudes towards pre-marital sex and single motherhood, resulted in a steady decline in the demand for places in the former Magdalen Homes. Within a few years, the institution had been largely consigned to history.

Chapter 20

Local Authority Children's Homes

The Local Government Act of 1929 brought a major new player into the children's care arena – the local authority. The Act, which came into effect on 1 April 1930, abolished boards of guardians and transferred the administration of poor relief (or public assistance, as it was now officially known) to county councils and county borough councils. In the case of some county councils, a single authority took over the duties previously performed by a dozen or more separate unions.

Despite this change of management, things by and large carried on much the same way as before. A few of the former workhouses were closed and the sites disposed of, particularly those in inconvenient locations or whose buildings were beyond redemption. Most, however, continued in use as council-run Public Assistance Institutions (PAIs), with exactly the same premises, staff and inmates as before. As if to emphasize the lack of change, the body set up to administer public assistance in each council area was usually known as the guardians' committee. Under council control, relatively little altered for the inmates of PAIs. The buildings sometimes saw some improvement, and inmates were allowed a little more freedom in going out or receiving visitors.

It was much the same story when it came to the councils' new responsibilities in the area of children's care. The residential facilities that they inherited were largely carried on as before, except for some rationalization of the accommodation and disposal of property that was deemed unsuitable or deemed surplus to requirements. In the first five years of the new arrangements, 120 council-run homes were closed.[1] Relatively few new children's establishments were opened by local authorities in the 1930s.

Like the boards of guardians before them, councils made use of boarding out. This could either be with a foster family or in one of the many voluntary homes certified for the purpose, the latter option being a useful way of dealing with fluctuations in demand. Some of the voluntary homes also provided facilities for children with particular needs, such as those with physical or mental problems. On the whole, though, the use of boarding out by local authorities during this period was relatively limited, at least in England and Wales. Institutional care of the young, which – despite government criticism – sometimes still took place in PAIs, was often a cheaper option. Not all children were considered suitable for boarding out – it was common practice that only children who were considered physically and mentally fit would be placed with foster parents. Non-white and older children often proved difficult to place. The need for good monitoring and supervision of children in foster care also provided a deterrent to its greater uptake. Much more enthusiasm for boarding out was, however, found in Scotland where in 1945 more than two-thirds of children in council care were being boarded out.[2]

The Second World War

The Second World War was a period of intense debate about the provision of welfare in Britain, with the 1942 Beveridge Report providing a blue-print for what was to become known as the welfare state. A number of other events were to have a particular influence on the reform of child care.

In 1939–40, over a million mainly working-class children from towns and cities considered to be at risk from enemy bombing were evacuated to the countryside to live with foster families. Their hosts, who were frequently middle class, often had to cope with difficulties such as head lice, bed-wetting, unhealthy feeding habits and bad manners from the new arrivals. The exercise did, however, greatly increase the awareness of the poor conditions in which many city children lived. In 1943, the Women's Group on Public Welfare published its influential book *Our Towns: A Close-Up*, based on a survey of evacuees and their foster carers. The Group's chair, Margaret Bondfield, made a plea for the building of 'a co-ordinated structure of services which leaves no gap. Education – physical, mental and social – must be the birthright of all.'[3]

Another influential children's welfare campaigner was Lady Marjory Allen. In a letter to *The Times* on 15 July 1944, she contended that in many 'Homes' the staff, though willing, were generally overworked, underpaid and untrained. The official inspection of establishments was also totally inadequate. She ended by calling for a public inquiry to ascertain whether public and charitable organizations were, in fact, enabling children to lead full and happy lives. Her letter provoked an enormous response.

The subject of fostering was put under the spotlight following the death in January 1945, of 13-year-old Dennis O'Neill. Dennis and his two younger brothers had been taken into local authority care in 1939 and boarded out in a succession of foster homes. He had finally ended up on a remote farm in Minsterly in Shropshire where he was beaten and starved by his foster father. Following an inquest, which criticized the local authority's lack of supervision, and an inquiry chaired by Sir William Monckton, an official committee was appointed, under Miss Myra Curtis, 'to inquire into the existing methods of providing for children who ... are deprived of a normal home life with their own parents or relatives; and to consider what further measures should be taken to ensure that these children are brought up under conditions best calculated to compensate them for the lack of parental care'.[4]

The Curtis Report

The Curtis Committee met for sixty-four days, heard 229 witnesses, and visited 451 institutions across England and Wales where children were being maintained. The Committee's report, published in 1946, noted a wide variation in the conditions they had encountered. Although many establishments were good, the worst left a great deal to be desired. In one former workhouse

> the Matron had made a valiant attempt to gather the children together in the most difficult circumstances. She had to use the institution kitchen as a dining room for the toddlers. We saw them just after the tables had been cleared at dinner time. Most of them had folded their arms on the table and were asleep, with their heads on their hands, while their feet swung aimlessly from a too high wooden bench. The kitchen fire provided warmth and comfort; compared with the cheerless and bare day room they were better off in the warm kitchen. They had large chipped enamel mugs to drink from, such as were familiar at one time in casual wards; we were told that casual wards are now supplied with crockery. At this institution the 'mother' in charge of the children was a harassed looking woman doing her best in difficult circumstances. The Master and Matron were young keen people suffering from a sense of frustration. The Matron complained about the seeming inertia of Public Assistance Committee members. It was noted that the chairman of the Public Assistance Committee was 91 and the Vice Chairman over 80. The impression was left that they were maintaining standards of 50 years ago.[5]

In some areas, it was clear that

> the workhouse served as a dumping ground for children who could
> not readily be disposed of elsewhere, and that in some districts where
> children's Homes provided insufficient accommodation, or boarding
> out had not been well developed, older children, for whom there had
> never been any properly planned accommodation, were looked after
> in the workhouse for a considerable length of time.[6]

A similar variation was found in the voluntary homes examined by the
Committee. This category included

> a large number of institutional Homes of the 'barrack' variety often with
> imposing buildings, built as a symbol of Victorian philanthropy and
> intended to catch the eye and to impress the passer by. In these Homes
> the rooms were often bare and comfortless, and so large that it was usu-
> ally impossible to set aside any place for quiet occupations or hobbies.[7]

Even where voluntary organizations housed their children in smaller
homes, the care within them varied widely. At one establishment, a
branch of a large voluntary organization,

> we saw a young foster mother and her assistant who were bringing
> up 20 little girls aged 5 to 14 in a pleasant villa on the outskirts of a
> large town. The Home looked much like other houses in the vicinity;
> there was nothing to distinguish it from its neighbours either by size
> or grounds. There was the usual tennis court and vegetable garden
> found attached to homes of this type. The House was not too large to
> be homely, and it was evident that it did represent home to the little
> girls who lived in it.[8]

In contrast, another house of a similar type was a picture of desolation:

> The place was rambling, inconvenient and incredibly bare. In the
> boys' rooms there was nothing to sit on and nothing to play with.
> Difficult as such a place must have been to use, it was not impossible
> and the plan of the building was such as to lend itself more readily to
> small sub-divisions than a more compact place. Nothing of this kind
> had, however, been tried and the boys lived, ate and slept in dormito-
> ries on much the same lines as a barrack home.[9]

In its conclusions, the Curtis Report recommended that for children without parents or a satisfactory home, adoption was the ideal

option, with fostering the next best alternative. If a child had to undergo institutional care, then this should be in small homes of ideally no more than eight children. Children in such homes should be encouraged to maintain contact with relatives and to develop friendships outside the home. Brothers and sisters in care should be kept together.

The Committee's endorsement of fostering was not entirely unequivocal, however. Its carefully worded judgement was that 'boarding out is to be preferred to institutional care for children who are suitable for boarding out'[10] and noted that 'that there is probably a greater risk of acute unhappiness in a foster home, but that a happy foster home is happier than life as generally lived in a large community'.[11] These caveats were largely ignored and fostering rapidly came to be seen as the favoured option for any child in need of a home.

The Clyde Report

In parallel with the work of the Curtis Committee, a similar review was carried out in Scotland with a senior Scottish judge, James Clyde, as its chair. The Clyde Report, which was also published in 1946, again laid a strong emphasis on foster care as providing the means by which a homeless child 'secures the necessary opportunity to build up its own personality and equip itself for the transition to independence and self-reliance'.[12] The Report recommended an expansion of fostering, with local authority children's committees having sole responsibility for deprived children. It also called for the end of placement of children in poorhouses, but recognized that there would still be a need for residential institutions for some children. Such homes, however, required improvement in matters such as their location, layout, maximum size, dietary provision and recreational facilities. After-care, too, needed to be accentuated.

The 1948 Children Act

The Curtis Report's proposals formed the basis of the 1948 Children Act which placed local authorities at the centre of an integrated system of child care service provision. The overall operation of the new system was placed under the supervision of the Home Office.

Under the Act, local authorities were given the duty of taking into their care children in their area, under the age of 17, a) who had no parent or guardian, or had been abandoned by them, or b) whose parents or guardian were unable, due to incapacity, to provide and care for them. In either case, the intervention of the local authority was required to be in what was judged to be the interests of the welfare of the child.

Voluntary homes still had their part to play in the new system but all now had to be registered with the Home Office and subject to official inspection. In return, however, they could receive government grants to improve their premises or improve staffing.

To fulfil their new obligations, local authorities were required to establish a Children's Committee and to appoint a children's officer to manage the practical implementation of the new system through the creation of a council Children's Department. Initially, councils faced a variety of difficulties in meeting these demands. The remit of the new scheme required the integration of activities previously divided between its health and education departments and public assistance committee, each of which had had their own policies and ways of working. Finding suitably qualified candidates for the new children's officer posts could prove difficult, particularly as most of these were expected to be women, who rarely had the senior management experience that was usually asked for. The councillors who sat on the new Children's Committees were not guaranteed to be supportive of the legislative changes that had taken place. The same could also be true for staff who were redeployed to work in the new Children's Departments, or who ran the council's existing residential homes and might be feeling anxious about their future.[13]

As the new structure settled into place, many of the new Children's Departments organized campaigns to recruit additional foster parents. In Birmingham, the council produced promotional pamphlets and its staff gave talks to many local groups. In 1951, cinemas in the area screened a Home Office film entitled *A Family Affair*, which aimed to encourage members of the public to offer foster homes, which was accompanied by lantern slides referring to the local need for homes and giving the address of the Children's Department. Not all offers of help could be used however, such as one in a letter which said, in effect, 'My wife is very neurotic and the doctor says a child would do her good. Can you please let us have one?'[14]

Despite the new emphasis of fostering, local authorities could still make use of measures such as adoption and even emigration in finding suitable homes for those coming into its care. The ability of an authority to place children for adoption was clarified as part of the 1949 Adoption Act.

Councils also continued to provide their own residential accommodation, both short term and longer term, for children that came into their care. Initially, much of this need was met by their existing stocks of property, most of which had been inherited in 1930 from the workhouse authorities. Many of these premises had originated as cottage homes and scattered homes and were on a scale which broadly fitted in with the Curtis Report's proposal that residential care should be in relatively small, family-style groups. This placed councils in a rather better situation than organizations in the voluntary sector, where many homes were located in large institutional buildings.

Throughout the 1950s and '60s, local authorities established a large number of new homes to either replace or supplement their existing children's accommodation. At the outset, they typically purchased existing houses – these were often quite substantial properties with ample gardens. By the mid-1950s, however, many urban councils were including children's homes in the large housing estates that they were erecting around their towns and cities. These 'family group homes', as they were now generally known, normally followed the scattered homes principle of being thinly distributed and were often indistinguishable from the ordinary houses around them, apart perhaps from being a slightly larger version.

In 1948, the Leeds City Council established its new Children's Committee, whose responsibilities had previously been spread across separate Health, Education and Social Welfare committees. In addition to two Approved Schools and a Remand Home, its housing stock at that date included two nurseries, seven children's homes ranging from a small home for eight girls to a mixed home accommodating fifty-six boys and girls, and a group of five cottage homes in Rothwell. Much of this had been inherited from the workhouse authorities in 1930 and virtually all these premises were now overcrowded, inadequate, and in need of repair and adaptation. Over the next eight years, a development programme resulted in the building of sixteen family group homes, each accommodating eight children, spread across the city's new housing estates. Four larger properties were also purchased, and a former 'central' home converted into a reception centre and short-stay home. The ageing Rothwell cottage homes, which had begun to be affected by mining subsidence, were closed.

In Manchester, the city's Children's Committee had inherited the children's cottage homes at Styal, erected in 1898 by the Chorlton Union.

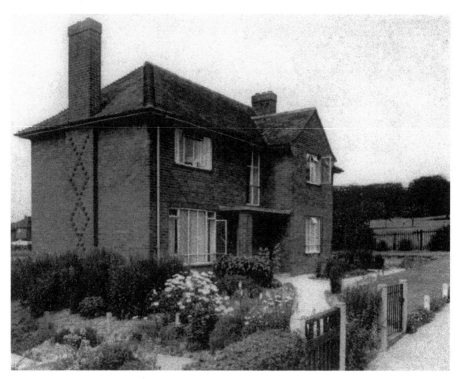

A family group home erected by Leeds City Council on one of its new housing estates in the early 1950s.

When they were closed in 1956, twenty-seven of the forty-six planned family group homes had been constructed on the Corporation's new housing estates. Of these, twenty-three were four-bedroomed houses each accommodating six children, and four were six-bedroomed houses each accommodating eight children. Most of the homes were staffed by married couples, some of whom had one or two children of their own. The husband followed his normal occupation and in return for his board, lodging, and allowance, devoted part of his leisure time to the children and to assisting his wife. Each housemother was encouraged to run her home as an ordinary mother would do. A part-time daily domestic who acted as relief for time off and for holidays was also employed in each home. The Committee's report for 1955/56 recorded that a coloured married couple had been appointed to look after a family of coloured children. It was also noted that many of the homes had made their own summer holiday arrangements, some going to the Isle of Man, others to the Yorkshire coast or to holiday camps. As well as the family group homes, the council operated a reception and observation centre, a residential nursery, two short-stay homes, two long-stay homes, two hostels, two Remand Homes and an Approved School. Of the 2,170 children in its care, 717 were boarded out or in residential employment or on trial with parents.[15]

Between 1952 and 1970, the national total of children in local authority care gradually rose from nearly 65,000 to just over 71,000, although this represented a fairly constant proportion of around 0.5 per cent of the nation's under-18s.[16] This was in spite of the 1963 Children and Young Persons Act introducing a duty for local authorities 'to promote the welfare of children by diminishing the need to receive or keep them in care'. Children's Departments were now expected to undertake preventive activities, for example by working with children and parents at home.

With Home Office encouragement, the proportion of children being boarded out by councils rose from around 41 per cent in 1952 to a peak of 48 per cent in 1963–4. However, it then fell back to just over 42 per cent in 1970, virtually its 1952 level. The reasons for this decrease are

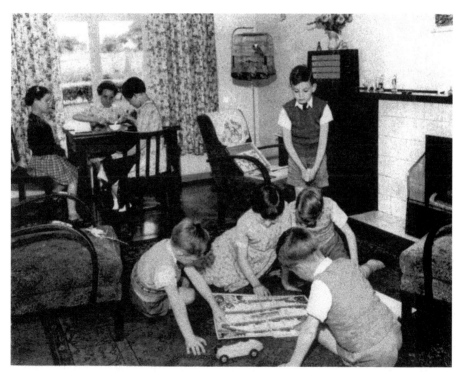

A cosy domestic scene in one of the Leeds Council's new children's homes, early 1950s

unclear. One factor was a decline in the supply of foster mothers in some parts of the country. According to a report published in 1957, three-fifths of the foster mothers surveyed were aged over 40 at the time of the child being placed with them. Half had no other child, and more than a third were childless. Almost none was in paid work and the majority were working class.[17] By the mid-1960s, however, there was an increasing trend for working-class wives to go out to work and the generally low payments offered for boarding out often compared badly with the wages that could be earned even in part-time employment. Another factor was the long-term nature of much fostering which reduced the possibility of using foster parents for a succession of different children.

In 1952, around 25 per cent of children boarded out by councils were placed in voluntary sector homes, a figure that had halved by 1961. During the following decade, the number gradually recovered, rising to almost 18 per cent by 1970.

A New Era

The 1969 Children and Young Persons Act proposed that an integrated network of Community Homes should be developed on a regional basis to replace the existing system of Approved Schools, Remand Homes, local authority children's homes and reception centres. Voluntary homes could also be incorporated into the new scheme either as Controlled Community Homes or Assisted Community Homes, according to whether the management, equipment and maintenance of the home was to be the prime responsibility of the local authority or of the voluntary organization. Those voluntary homes unable or unwilling to join in the new proposals could continue to operate under the existing arrangements for their regulation and inspection. Under the new scheme, most former Approved Schools were redesignated as Community Homes with Education, with many coming under council control for the first time.

Another upheaval was brought about by the 1970 Social Services Act which required local authorities to bring together their various social work and social care activities, including those for children, and to establish Social Services departments. The absorption of former Children's Departments into the new structure, and the resulting rationalization of staff, provided an unexpected bonus for the voluntary sector where many experienced child care workers found new employment.

The number of children in local authority accommodation now began to rise steeply, from 20,720 children in 1970 to its peak of 35,172 in 1976. Part of this increase was due to Community Homes with Education (the former Approved Schools) now being included in the figures. More significant, however, was the fact that more children were coming into care and were being retained longer in council-run homes. In 1974, a high-profile inquiry into the death of Maria Colwell at the hands of her stepfather concluded that co-ordination between child welfare services was seriously lacking – a criticism that no doubt resulted in the greater caution of councils in releasing children from their care. The increasing concern about child protection issues in the wake of the Maria Colwell case was apparent in the 1975 Children Act which made the welfare of the child paramount in all decisions about its future. The Act made it easier for a child to be adopted or be placed in long-term foster care, even if this was contrary to the parents' wishes. One casualty of this trend was the voluntary sector, where local authority placements fell from 5,480 in 1971 to 3,400 in 1978.

The 1970s witnessed a number of other changes that were to have a considerable impact on children's residential care. There was a move away from the joint appointment of married couples to run homes. This practice had sometimes caused difficulties through the demands from a couple's own children. There were also sometimes problems where the work of one of the pair was satisfactory but the other was not. The trend towards the professionalization of residential care staff led to their now being employed on individual contracts based on their particular qualifications and experience. The introduction of legal limits on the length of the working week meant that additional staff needed to be employed in order to provide cover on a shift system, and it was rarely possible for them to all be resident. There was a move in the late 1970s to charging residential workers market-related rents for their accommodation, with salaries being correspondingly increased. This made 'living-in' financially much less attractive than had previously been the case. Family group homes were increasingly recast as small group homes, staffed by a team of staff under the management of an officer in charge.

The 1980s saw a steady decline of the number of children in residential care – down to around 14,000 in 1987 compared to around 37,000 a decade earlier.[18] Apart from the increased emphasis on fostering, particularly long-term fostering, there was a decline in the number of older children in the general population – the group most likely to go into residential care. As a result, many local authorities began to reduce their stock of children's accommodation – a trend that was taken to its ultimate extent by Warwickshire County Council which, in 1986, closed the last of its own children's homes.

The Voluntary Homes Bow Out

The changes that were affecting local authorities had an even greater impact on the Community Homes run by the voluntary sector, where funding had always been precarious at the best of times. The increasing costs of running and staffing the homes, coupled with the steady decrease in demand for places, led many children's long-established organizations to call it a day. Some charities merged with one another, or simply decided to wind themselves up – perhaps converting their remaining assets into a grant-making trust. Others decided to keep going but to change their focus and direct their efforts into more specialist areas, for example, in providing services for children with special needs, or in supporting families in keeping children living at home. In some cases, voluntary bodies became suppliers of such services to local authorities, although this could be risky path – a council's spending priorities could easily change and contracts not be renewed, leaving the provider high and dry. By the end of the 1980s, however, it was clear that the long and hallowed tradition of 'general' children's homes being run by charitable bodies had come to an end.

In more recent times, the growing presence of the commercial sector in health and social care provision has been particularly evident in the market for children's residential facilities. In 2000, the number of privately run homes in England was just two hundred and fifty-six. By 2014, the number had risen to 1,293, accounting for 73 per cent of the national total, while those run by voluntary bodies made up only 6 per cent. Local authorities, a third of whom no longer had a council-run children's home, contributed the remaining 21 per cent.[19]

Chapter 21

Life in Children's Homes

What was life like for children in residential care? There is no simple answer to this question – it varied considerably according to the period under consideration, the type of institution and the individual staff who ran a particular institution.

Views about how children should be treated have evolved considerably over the years. The Victorian era is often characterized by popular expressions of the period such as 'Children should be seen and not heard' or 'Spare the rod and spoil the child', with discipline, education, religious instruction and training for future employment seen as the key components of a life in a children's home. Corporal punishment, for boys at least, was commonplace. These attitudes applied more or less equally to those in residence at expensive public schools and to those in establishments run by charities or by the Poor Law authorities.

First-hand descriptions of life for children in residential institutions come from a variety of sources. Those involved in the running of the establishments invariably presented them in glowing terms. A typical report was given by a 'visitor' to the Waifs and Strays Society home at Cullercoats, Northumberland, in 1892:

> At 6 a.m. a bell rings to awaken the household. Each one is expected to rise at once. The 'house girls' then went off to their work, and the 'laundry girls' to theirs; and all this was so quietly and gently performed that, if I had not been listening, I should not have heard the least sound.
>
> At 7.30 a.m. the bell sounds again, and the large family of 40 girls, aged from 4 to 16 years, begin to assemble in the large dining room for breakfast. The girls are all seated round one long table, and are now eagerly eating their porridge and bread and milk. As the children filed into the room, there was a general morning salutation, and the gentle curtsey dropped. None could doubt that the lady superintendent was loved and respected, and that she was a mother among them all. All her plans, though very simple in their character, were orderly, methodical, and regular, and each member of family seemed to take a pleasure in fulfilling wishes, and doing all in their power to prove that the confidence placed in them was not misjudged.

*After breakfast all proceeded to the little chapel where matins was sung,
the children all taking part in a very bright intelligent manner, and their
voices blending in earnest joyous praise in the two hymns they sang.*[1]

Rather more down to earth was the account by an assistant house-
mother of the usual day at Barnardo's Boys Garden City, Woodford
Bridge, in the 1920s. At 6 a.m., the 'house boy' – a 14-year-old who had
left school – rose to light the kitchen and sitting-room fires, scrub the
kitchen floor etc. After being woken at 6.30, the other boys dressed,
stripped their beds and turned their mattresses, then had prayers on
the landing before doing housework until 7.30. Boots were cleaned
and the boys strip-washed in a cold wash-house with cold water. After
being inspected they marched to the central dining-hall for breakfast.
After school, plenty of outdoor activities were available and swimming was much encouraged.[2]

Helping with the household chores was something that both boys
and girls were expected to do and in some types of establishment, such
as Industrial Schools, virtually all the housework, cooking and laundry
was carried out by the inmates. As well as learning skills such sewing
and cooking, boys would also undertake the heavier jobs, such as chopping firewood or carrying water. For the girls, such work would be part
of their preparation for employment in domestic service which, up until
the First World War at least, was their most likely future occupation.

The food provided at children's homes – as in many ordinary British
households of the time – was invariably fairly plain. At the NCH's
Newton Hall home in Cheshire, breakfast consisted of bread and milk
or porridge and a mug of cocoa. Dinner offerings included stew, fish
or cold meat and vegetables followed by rice pudding or 'figgy duff'.
For tea, there was bread and margarine with jam or golden syrup and
a mug of cocoa, with a cake or bun and weak tea on Sundays. A breakfast treat on Good Friday was a boiled or poached egg and a toasted
bun, while birthdays were celebrated with a small sausage roll.[3]

The predictability of the weekly routine in many homes could be
oppressive. According to one Waifs and Strays inmate: 'Of the meals,
I can only remember boiled liver on Thursdays, fish on Fridays.'[4]
Another recalled: 'Tuesday evening it was stocking mending time, we
all sat round the dining room table … in dead silence, not a word must
be spoken, and whoever got theirs done first had to do the younger
children's, as you may imagine we didn't hurry too much.'[5]

The imposition of silence was not uncommon. At the Waifs and
Strays Home at Longwell Green, near Bristol, silence was required

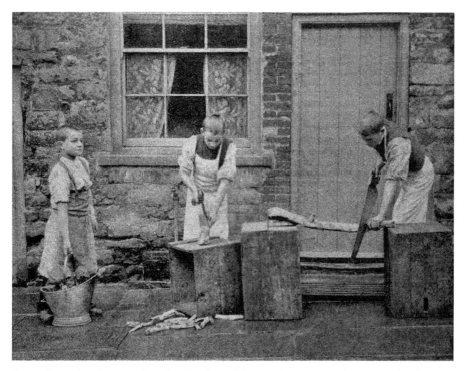

Boys chopping firewood at the Waifs and Strays Society home at Lincoln, 1890s.

virtually the whole time except for quiet conversation between tea and bedtime. At the Hull home, the whole of Good Friday had to be spent in silence. At Dover in 1902, Sunday mornings were spent at church and Sunday School, while the afternoons were spent sitting round the dining room in complete silence with no books or games. The house-mother would occasionally peep round the door and any boy caught so much as smiling would be caned.[6] A common Friday night ritual was the dosing the children with an 'opening' mixture such as brimstone and treacle, or castor-oil and powdered liquorice.

At the Nazareth House home for girls in Newcastle, the weekly Friday night bath was a complicated affair due to modesty needing to be preserved at all times. Each girl's bath, supervised by a senior girl, took place in a cubicle while wearing a heavy bath-sheet with arm holes in it. Washing was with carbolic soap and the same water was used for a number of girls.[7] At the same institution, the children were addressed by their allocated number rather than their surname – a practice which continued until after the Second World War.[8] The same custom pertained at the Southampton Union cottage homes.

At many institutions, the punishments dealt out to miscreants would now be viewed as cruel and degrading. In Reformatories, Industrial Schools and workhouses, flogging was the standard punishment for boys who committed serious misdemeanours. Although its use in workhouses was covered by detailed regulations – for example, that a beating could only take place after two hours had elapsed since the offence for which it was being administered – the rules were not always adhered to. In 1847, a 5-year-old orphan, later to become famous as Henry Morton Stanley, the journalist who tracked down Dr Livingstone, became an inmate of the St Asaph workhouse in North Wales. The scourge of the workhouse was its schoolmaster, James Francis, whose cruelty seemed to know no bounds. In 1856, after a scratch had been made on a new table, Francis began to birch every boy in the class until the culprit confessed. When Stanley's turn came, his accumulated rage finally boiled over, he knocked out the teacher and escaped from the workhouse.

Rather more typical was the story of George Poole who, at the end of the First World War, was an inmate of a home in Coventry which housed thirty boys aged from 3 to 14 years. The staff consisted of a matron and two assistants. He recalled:

> We used to get up early each morning and do certain tasks such as make our own beds the uniform way, to clean or scrub floors. Then we had to get ourselves washed for school and parade for inspection. If any of these duties were not performed correctly punishment was given, such as the birch or belt across the bare bottom or the hairbrush on the back of the hand. The worst example was when a boy of three years old soiled his trousers: the matron paraded all us boys in the yard to witness her throwing a cold bucket of water over him naked. I know what the hairbrush punishment was like. She gave it to me for something I didn't do which still sticks in my memory. It left lumps on my hands for a month.[9]

There were also, of course, happy times for children in care. Christmas was always a special occasion, with local well-wishers often providing special donations or other contributions. Homes would be decorated, a Christmas tree put up and a stocking filled with small gifts for each child. Food on Christmas day would include a festive dinner and treats such as nuts, dates, apples, oranges, biscuits and sweets. Afterwards there might be singing, games and other entertainment such as a magic lantern show. In some towns, local theatres would invite children from local homes to a performance of the annual pantomime. Some homes even mounted their own theatrical or musical shows.

In the summer, seaside outings became common, either as a day-trip or as a stay of up to several weeks. Some Waifs and Strays branches organized exchanges with one another, typically with a home located in a town or city swapping premises with one in the countryside or by the sea. In 1921, the girls from the Society's home in Brighton did an exchange with their counterparts at the St Hilda's Home in Beckenham. All their luggage was packed up in a large van for the trip. A few homes also had their own holiday home where groups of children could spend time. In 1925, the Leeds Catholic Diocese Rescue Society acquired a property in the countryside at Boston Spa, for use as a holiday home for girls from St Mary's Orphanage in Leeds. Many homes, particularly those for boys, used camping as an economical way of giving the children a holiday.

Other small treats could include a modest weekly hand-out of pocket money to buy sweets at a local shop. Children in some homes could look forward to a weekly outing to a Saturday morning cinema show.

Many homes allowed the keeping of pets for the children's interest and enjoyment. These could be communal animals such as a dog or a

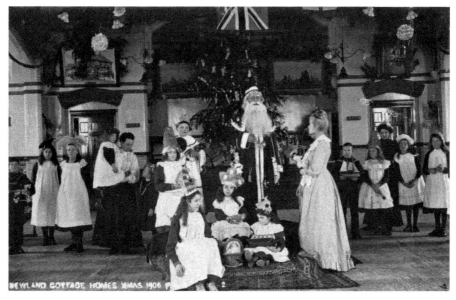

Christmas festivities at the Sailors' Orphan Homes (also known as the Newland Cottage Homes), in Hull in about 1905.

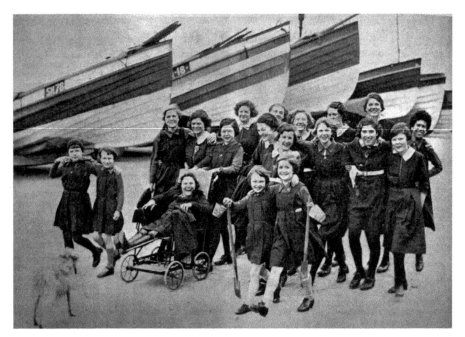

Girls from the St Chad's Waifs and Strays Society home, Leeds, on a seaside outing to Filey in around 1935.

baby goat, or individual ones such as guinea pigs, rabbits, hamsters and canaries. At the Waifs and Strays Society home in Wrexham, the boys kept pet jackdaws. In the 1920s, the Society's home for disabled children in Pyrford had a donkey which, as well as being a pet for the children, helped carry heavy items such as baskets of laundry or buckets of water.

After the Second World War, change was in the air. Many former single-sex establishments became mixed, the change being accompanied by an alteration of name such as Barnardo's girls' home in Barkingside becoming the Children's Village Home. In 1946, the Curtis Report had endorsed boarding out over institutional care which, if necessary, should only be in small family-style groups. For the Waifs and Strays Society, renamed the Church of England Children's Society in the same year, this did not present too great a challenge. Its homes had generally been modest in size – typically from twenty to thirty children – and it had always viewed fostering as the ideal form of care.

Organizations which housed children in large, old buildings faced a bigger challenge. One solution, which was the path followed by the Shaftesbury Homes, was to sell off some of these properties and replace them by smaller and more modern buildings. In some cases, large institutions tried to reconfigure their accommodation to support family groups. At the Actors' Orphanage, for example, large dormitories were partitioned into single-occupancy cubicles and the children formed into smaller groups which were each placed under the care of house-parents. In 1959, after adapting its premises, the NCH's Newton Hall home laid claim to being the organization's first property to consist entirely of mixed family groups of eight children. For charities such as Barnardo's, though, burdened by a large portfolio of often dilapidated properties, an antiquated administration and a shortage of funds, it took a long time to adjust to the new climate.

For local authorities, who were less hampered by the weight of tradition in their newly enlarged responsibilities towards the care of children, and financially better placed, change came more readily. In 1953, the Children's Committee of Birmingham City Council reported on the alterations that had been introduced over the previous four years at its Shenley Fields cottage homes site. The titles of Superintendent and Matron had been abolished from day to day use, as had the wearing of uniforms other than in the sick bay. The system of housing the children in groups according to their age had been dropped and a child now stayed in the same house for their entire stay, with brothers and sisters now able to live together. Girls reaching employment age were no longer transferred to live in a hostel but could go out to work from their existing home. No religious services were now held on the site. Children were encouraged to join life in the outside community such as youth clubs, scouts, guides and brownies, units of the Sea Scouts and St John Ambulance Brigade, a nearby athletics club, classes at an Evening Institute, ice-skating in Birmingham, train-spotting outings and trips to theatres, exhibitions and football matches. Financial support was given to excursions originated by the children themselves – this had included one boy's trip to London by himself. Cycling was also popular, with the homes having a pool of bicycles for use on a rota system. In 1952, a party of five girls had gone youth-hostelling, and a group of children went camping most weekends.[10]

Some homes run by religious groups were also undergoing transformation, as recalled by an inmate of the Nazareth House in Newcastle:

> *Great changes took place between 1946 and 1947. Sister Pauline's regimentation became more relaxed. Instead of long crocodiles of children, we were put into teams or what was known as Houses.*

Red, yellow, blue and green. We sported our tin-plate, brightly coloured badges on our gym tunics and wore them with pride. Even the napkin rings in the refectory were changed from the nondescript bone colour to brilliantly coloured house colours. Accomplishment awards were given out and there were goals to be achieved ... Our much loved chaplain, Father Cronin, started a theatre group; we put on plays and school concerts were performed ... A classroom, no longer in use, was turned miraculously into a common room furnished with lovely bright chintz-covered easy chairs and a piano was installed for the children to play. Quite a change from the austere, clinical and emotionally sterile regimented atmosphere of days gone by.[11]

Even Barnardo's was slowly coming to terms with the changing world. Its internal rule book for staff was updated in 1955 and the superintendents of its homes were exhorted to 'use their imagination and sympathy to realize what it must feel like to a child to be separated from all it has known ... There must be warmth in the welcome, friendliness, informality and understanding. The child should be allowed to retain his own possessions and the comfort of all possible links with home.'[12] By the 1960s, getting-up time in Barnardo homes was now usually no earlier than 7 a.m. Except for small tasks such as laying tables and washing up, the daily housework was done by cleaners. Children received pocket money that was comparable to that given by most parents, and increased with age. From the age of 12, children received their own monthly clothing allowance, then between fifteen and thirty shillings a month. This was not given in cash but its value could be used at a local store, such as Marks and Spencer, where the home had an account.[13]

According to a study of children's homes in the 1990s, those housing adolescents were often very quiet during the day, with few of the inmates attending school. After getting up late, they mysteriously disappeared 'supposedly to visit relatives but more probably to hang around the local shopping centre. Others sat watching television or accompanied staff on errands.'[14] Although shift rotas meant that children sometimes had a multiplicity of staff looking after them, there was often a great camaraderie between children and their carers, particularly in the evenings when outings might be organized, or the cooking of unhealthy treats take place in the home's kitchen.

Chapter 22

Abuse in Children's Homes

Over the past few years, the image of many once-hallowed children's institutions has been greatly tarnished by revelations of the serious physical and sexual abuse that went on behind their doors and, in some cases, the cover-ups that took place when such events became known to those in charge.

The abuse of children by those into whose care they had been placed is not, however, an exclusively modern phenomenon. In Victorian times, there were a number of well-publicized incidents, particularly in relation to workhouse inmates. In 1841, G. R. Wythen Baxter published *The Book of the Bastiles* – a compilation of newspaper reports, court proceedings, correspondence and other material that graphically illustrated some of the alleged horror stories relating to the New Poor Law. A typical item is given below:

> *An inquiry has taken place this week at Rochester, before the county magistrates, into several charges preferred against James Miles, the master of the Hoo Union-House, for cruelly beating several young pauper-children of both sexes. Elizabeth Danes stated that she was 13 years of age, and that the defendant, James Miles, had punished her three times while she was in the Union-House. The offence she had committed was leaving a little dirt in the corner of a room, and the defendant made her lie upon a table, and took her clothes off, and beat her with a birch-broom until blood came.*[1]

In 1894, Ella Gillespie, a nurse at the Hackney workhouse school at Brentwood, was accused of systematic cruelty to the children in her charge including beating them with stinging nettles and forcing them to kneel on wire netting that covered the hot water pipes. Children were also deprived of water and resorted to drinking from the toilet bowls. Her most notorious practice was night-time 'basket drill' where children were woken from their sleep and made to walk around the dormitory for an hour with a basket on their heads containing their day clothes, and receiving a beating if they dropped anything. After a trial for ill-treatment of children, Gillespie was sentenced to five years' penal servitude.[2]

In 1914, the Little Commonwealth, an experimental self-governing co-educational community, was founded in Evershot, Dorset. Run by Homer Lane, who had pioneered a similar scheme in America, it took children of all ages, including 'delinquents', and became a Certified Industrial School. The establishment closed in 1918 after Lane was accused of engaging in immoral relations with some of the girls.

In the 1920s, there were discussions in the medical literature concerning the appearance of venereal diseases such as gonorrhoea in babies and children resident in children's homes. A variety of explanations were put forward, such as infection from shared towels or lavatory seats, or sexual assault prior to entry to a home. However, it was apparently unthinkable that it could be caused through sexual abuse by an adult within the institution.[3]

Many cases of assault and other offences involving children in care were undoubtedly hushed up, but they did occasionally reach the courts. In July 1955, the Sheffield Corporation's Children's Officer, Ernest Healey, was sentenced to twelve months in prison for the indecent assault of three girls aged from 12 to 16. At least one of the incidents had taken place at the city's Grove Children's Home.[4]

Since the 1970s, an increasing volume of allegations of abuse from the former residents of children's homes, and the resulting inquiries, have led to an increasing realization of the scale of such activities.

Cosham Cottage Homes

Some of the victims of abuse have published personal memoirs detailing their experiences. Among these is the account by Les Cummings of growing up in the 1950s at the Cosham cottage homes run by Portsmouth City Council.[5] He and other inmates were frequently subjected by the staff to brutal violence and there were also several incidents of sexual impropriety. On one occasion, two boys were wrongly accused of having caused the death of two birds by raiding their nests for eggs. As a punishment, the homes' deputy superintendent forced the birds' bodies into the boys' mouths. Even worse, however, was the time Les spent with council-appointed foster parents where he was regularly beaten, starved and sexually abused. Despite making complaints to his placement officer, no action resulted. In 2006, then aged 62, Les demanded an apology from the council. This was refused, but following a radio programme about the homes in 2008, the council – though still not admitting liability – paid nineteen claimants a total of £92,000. In 2014, after a change in council leadership, the authority finally made a public apology for its failings. After examining allegations against the homes, the Crown Prosecution Service decided not to prosecute as seventeen of the alleged abusers had died and there was insufficient evidence against the remaining three.[6]

Kincora

The Kincora Hostel for Working Boys on Upper Newtownards Road, Belfast, was opened in 1958 by the Eastern Board of Northern Ireland. It accommodated boys of working age who had difficult home circumstances. On 24 January 1980, the *Irish Independent* newspaper reported that allegations of sexual abuse at the home had been made over a period of several years but no action had been taken. A few months later, three staff at the home were convicted of the systematic sexual abuse of inmates and given prison sentences ranging from four to six years. The home was then closed down.

Kincora has since been surrounded by claims of a cover-up by the Royal Ulster Constabulary linked to the alleged involvement of high-ranking civil servants and military officers in the abuse that took place. It was also claimed that one of the staff convicted, William McGrath, was an MI5 informer.

Pindown

One of the first major abuse investigations in England in modern times was into the practice of 'Pindown', employed at several children's homes run Staffordshire County Council between 1983 and 1989. Pindown – solitary confinement, for continuous periods of up to three months, clothed in pyjamas – was used as a punishment for behaviour such as absconding, theft or bullying. After its use came to light in September 1989, enormous public concern was expressed and taken up by the media. The following June, Staffordshire Council appointed Allan Levy QC and Barbara Kahan, Chair of the National Children's Bureau, to conduct an independent inquiry into the use of Pindown. They concluded that Pindown 'contained the worst elements of institutional control'. For those undergoing the regime, it was a 'narrow, punitive and harshly restrictive experience' whose use resulted in despair, isolation, boredom, frustration and humiliation.[7] There was particular criticism for the council's Social Services Department, who appeared to be in ignorance of the use of Pindown in several of their children's homes, and of the system's instigator, Tony Latham, who despite his claimed positive intentions for the regime, had lost sight of the required standards of behaviour and professional practice.

Following the Pindown scandal, Sir William Utting was commissioned in 1991 to conduct a general review of children's residential care. His report made a number of recommendations aimed at improving staff selection and training.[8]

Leicestershire Council Homes

In November 1991, a former Royal Marine named Frank Beck was found guilty on seventeen counts involving sexual and physical assault on children at three Leicestershire Council children's homes where he was superintendent between 1973 and 1986. He was given five life sentences.

It was revealed that following an anonymous complaint in 1975 about the treatment of children at Beck's establishment, then located at Ratcliffe Road, Leicester, he had been called before a meeting of the council but managed to persuade them to endorse his approach. Despite a number of complaints subsequently being made, including several to the police, none resulted in any proceedings against Beck or his colleagues until 1989 when the investigation began that was to lead to his conviction.

In 1992, following the Beck trial, two inquiries were launched. The first, led by Andrew Kirkwood QC, examined the circumstances surrounding the events at the council's homes. It found that Beck – a charismatic and physically powerful character – had instituted a regime where children were encouraged to regress temporarily to an early stage in their development. This involved a considerable degree of personal physical contact with staff, including hugging and firm holding.

Kirkwood's report also noted that the 1970s had seen 'a deliberate move away from the traditional arrangement whereby children's homes were in the hands of a husband and wife team as superintendent and matron, or officer in charge and deputy'.[9] Kirkwood suggested several reasons for this trend. Such joint appointments were increasingly regarded as 'collusive' because if problems occurred, a husband and wife would always back each other up. Furthermore, the appointment of a husband and wife to the two senior posts in a home led to rostering problems since both would want the same time off duty, with the home then being left in the charge of a junior employee. The increase in numbers of difficult adolescents then coming into the homes was viewed as needing a change from the 'Uncle and Auntie' style of leadership to one that was controlling but lively and imaginative.[10]

The second inquiry, chaired by Sir Norman Warner, looked at the recruitment, selection, appointment and supervision of staff in children's homes nationally. His report found that inadequate attention was being given to these matters by senior staff, and that workers were frequently being appointed who lacked adequate qualifications or experience.[11]

North Wales

What became known as the North Wales child abuse scandal began to surface in 1986 when allegations were made by Alison Taylor concerning the physical and sexual abuse of children by staff at a number of residential homes in the region. Taylor was then the Officer in Charge at the Ty Newydd children's home in Bangor, North Wales, run by the Gwynedd County Council. Her allegations were based on complaints from children coming to Ty Newydd from other establishments, both privately operated homes and ones run by Clywd and Gwynedd County Councils.

Taylor initially presented a dossier of the allegations to her council superiors but, after no action resulted, she went to the police, upon which the council suspended her. After an initial police investigation that also led to no proceedings being taken, Taylor was branded by the council as a 'blatant trouble maker' and 'a most unfit person to be in charge of a children's home'.[12] Undaunted, she continued her campaign for a public inquiry, unearthing further cases of abuse, including some by staff at the Clwyd Council's Bryn Estyn home in Wrexham. Following a major investigation by the North Wales Police during 1991–3, six individuals, including a deputy principal and a housemaster at Bryn Estyn, were convicted of serious sexual offences.

In 1994, Clywd Council commissioned John Jillings to chair an internal investigation into allegations of abuse against residents of its children's homes in the 1970s and 1980s. His report was completed two years later but not published because of legal advice that it could expose the authority to compensation claims from those involved.

In 1996, with ongoing public concern about child care in North Wales, William Hague, the then Secretary of State for Wales, ordered a judicial inquiry into the abuse of children in care homes in the former county council areas of Clwyd and Gwynedd (both authorities being abolished in 1996). A retired High Court judge, Sir Ronald Waterhouse, was appointed as its chair.

The Waterhouse Inquiry's findings, entitled *Lost in Care*, were published in February 2000. The report's major conclusion was that 'widespread sexual abuse of boys occurred in children's residential establishments in Clwyd between 1974 and 1990'.[13] The report provided an extensive catalogue of the offenders and offences. As well as Bryn Estyn, considerable abuse had occurred at the council's Cartrefle home in Broughton. There were some incidents of sexual abuse of girl residents in these establishments but they were comparatively rare.

The report also found that widespread sexual abuse of boys had taken place in privately run children's homes in Clwyd throughout the same period, with sexual abuse of girls also occurring to an alarming extent.[14] Prominent among these were the homes and hostels operated by the Bryn Alyn Community. In 1995, John Allen, the founder of the Community, was sentenced to six years' imprisonment for having sexually abused boys in his care during the 1970s. It also emerged that another member of the staff had been convicted in 1976 for sexual assaults on boys, and the deputy head teacher of the Community's school had been given six months' imprisonment in 1986 for unlawful sexual intercourse with a girl resident under 16 years of age.

As regards physical abuse, the Waterhouse Inquiry also revealed that unacceptable use of force in disciplining and restraining residents had occurred at not less than six local authority homes in Clwyd, despite Clwyd Council policy that no member of staff should inflict corporal punishment on any child or young person in any circumstances. The inquiry found that although some instances of abuse had taken place in Gwynedd, it had been on a very much smaller scale than in Clwyd.

Waterhouse concluded that no evidence had been presented to establish that there was a wide-ranging conspiracy involving prominent persons and others with the objective of sexual activity with children in care. It did accept, however, that a paedophile ring had operated in the Chester and Wrexham areas for much of the period under review.

The inquiry's seventy-two recommendations covered changes and improvements in areas such as the detection of, and response to, abuse, the prevention of abuse, the regulation of private homes, inspection procedures, the structure and training of staff and the consideration of strategic issues.

In 2013, a redacted version of the Jillings Report was finally released. It recorded: 'Our investigations have led us to conclude that the abuse of children and young people in Clwyd residential units has been extensive, and has taken place over a substantial number of years ... It is clear that, in a significant number of cases, the lives of young people who have been through the care system in Clwyd have been severely disrupted and disturbed. At least twelve young people are dead.'[15] Jillings severely criticized the North Wales Police, and noted that 'the most striking fact to emerge is that five men who shared in common their employment as residential care workers at Bryn Estyn were convicted of serious offences involving at least twenty-four young people'.[16]

Following the death of the television personality Jimmy Savile in 2011, a considerable number of allegations began to emerge about his abusive activities over a period of many years in a large number of institutions. These included a number of fresh complaints about abuse in homes in North Wales. In November 2012, the Prime Minister announced that a review would take place into the workings of the Waterhouse Inquiry, with Mrs Justice Julia Macur subsequently appointed to the task. At around the same time, a new investigation known as Operation Pallial was set up to examine the new and existing complaints. In August 2013, John Allen, now aged 71, appeared in court charged with thirty-two serious sexual offences relating to allegations of historic child abuse. He was later sentenced to life imprisonment.

Cyril Smith

As well as abuse at children's homes carried out by their own members of staff, an increasing number of cases have emerged of such crimes being committed by outsiders visiting these establishments on some pretext. A large number of Jimmy Savile's assaults were committed in hospitals and residential homes to which he had been a welcomed guest. Many similar allegations of sexual abuse have also emerged relating to other figures in the worlds of politics, entertainment and the media. Recent investigations into these events have invariably revealed a long history of complaints by the victims having been disbelieved, ignored or covered up.

Particularly shocking was the case of Cyril Smith, the Liberal MP for Rochdale between 1972 and 1992, who died in 2010. In 1968, a former inmate of Cambridge House, a boys' hostel in Rochdale founded by Smith, complained to the police about having been assaulted by Smith but was told he was 'a very important, powerful man'.[17]

Many further complaints were made over the years, particularly in relation to activities at Knowl View – a council-run special school for 8- to 16-year-olds with learning difficulties. The school, of which Smith was a governor and to which he owned a set of keys, was said to be a centre of paedophile activity involving Smith himself and many others outside. The worrying state of the school was described in a 1991 report to the Rochdale Council by its HIV Protection Officer, Phil Shepherd, and which was only released by the council, in redacted form, in 2014.[18] No action appears to have resulted from the report.

During his lifetime, Smith was interviewed by police on a number of occasions regarding allegations against him of sexual abuse or the possession of child pornography, but in each case he was quickly and mysteriously released, with no formal proceedings ensuing. According to one former Special Branch officer with the Lancashire Police, a dossier of allegations by boys claiming that they had been abused by Smith was suddenly removed to London by MI5 and no charges ever arose from it.[19]

Since Rochdale MP Simon Danczuk published a book about Smith's activities in 2014[20] there has been increasing speculation about the existence of a network of highly placed paedophiles at Westminster in which Smith was involved.

Events in the Rochdale homes are included among the investigations to be undertaken by the Independent Inquiry into Child Sexual Abuse (see following).

Irish Child Abuse Commission

In 1999, in the wake of a number of legal actions brought by former inmates of children's institutions in the country, the Irish government established the Commission to Inquire into Child Abuse. Its remit was to investigate the abuse of children in institutions in the State, primarily Reformatory and Industrial, Schools, between 1936 and the present time. These institutions were run by Roman Catholic religious orders such as the Irish Christian Brothers and the Sisters of Mercy.

The inquiry received harrowing details of practices that had been followed at various institutions. Typical was St Patrick's Industrial School in Upton, County Cork, owned and managed by the Rosminian Order. Seven sexual abusers were identified as having worked at the School, with at least three of them there at the same time in the 1950s. Those who were discovered had usually been transferred to other institutions.[21] Excessive physical punishment 'was an everyday occurrence and was brutal and severe'.[22] The general state of the School was also very poor. Following a visit in 1965, the Lord Mayor of Cork had expressed the opinion that the conditions he had witnessed 'would not be tolerated in a workhouse of by-gone days'.[23]

The Commission's report, published in 2009, contained forty-three conclusions, the first of which was that, 'Physical and emotional abuse and neglect were features of the institutions. Sexual abuse occurred in many of them, particularly boys' institutions. Schools were run in a severe, regimented manner that imposed unreasonable and oppressive discipline on children and even on staff.'[24] The report proposed twenty-one measures aimed at addressing the effects of the abuse on those who suffered, and to prevent or reduce the incidence of abuse of children in institutions. The recommendations included a proposal for the construction of a public memorial to abuse victims bearing the words of a statement made by the Taoiseach in May 1999: 'On behalf of the State and of all citizens of the State, the Government wishes to make a sincere and long overdue apology to the victims of childhood abuse for our collective failure to intervene, to detect their pain, to come to their rescue.'[25]

Jersey

In 2006, the States of Jersey Police began an investigation, later dubbed Operation Rectangle, into allegations of the abuse of children in care that had taken place on the island from the 1960s onwards. Evidence from witnesses increasingly placed the focus on a home known as Haut de la Garenne, which had begun life in 1867 as a boys' Industrial School, subsequently becoming known as the Jersey Home for Boys. In 1960, it merged with the Jersey Home for Girls and adopted the name Haut de la Garenne. The home finally closed in 1986. In February 2008, excavations at the site unearthed what were initially thought to be skull fragments although subsequent forensic analysis suggested they were more likely to be wood or coconut shell.

In March 2008, Jimmy Savile began legal proceedings against the *Sun* newspaper for linking him to the abuse at Haut de la Garenne. He claimed he had never visited the place, but later admitted having done so after a photograph emerged of him at the home surrounded by children.

In 2009 and 2010 a number of individuals were convicted of child abuse offences. These included Michael Aubin, for acts of gross indecency and indecent assault on children under the age of 10, committed while he himself was a child resident of Haut de la Garenne; Gordon

Wateridge, for acts of indecent assault and gross indecency while employed as house parent at Haut de la Garenne in the 1970s; and a married couple, Morag and Anthony Jordan, for physical abuse also while working as house parents in the 1970s.

Other complaints by former inmates about the treatment they received, such as being made to take cold showers, being slapped about the head, or flicked with a wet towel, were deemed not to warrant court proceedings.

In 2013, following continued complaints about police handling of the investigations, the States announced the setting up of the Independent Jersey Care Inquiry which began its hearings in July 2014. The inquiry, chaired by Frances Oldham QC, promised that it would conduct a robust and fearless examination of what went wrong and find answers for people who suffered abuse as children. The inquiry was expected to report its findings at the end of 2016.

Northern Ireland Historical Institutional Abuse Inquiry

In 2012, the Northern Ireland Assembly decided to follow the example of the Republic and establish its own Historical Institutional Abuse Inquiry (HIAI). The inquiry examined thirteen Catholic, secular, local authority and juvenile detention institutions in Northern Ireland covering the period from 1922 to 1995.

At an HIAI hearing on 12 February 2014, the inquiry heard that girls at the Londonderry Nazareth House had sometimes been punished by being bathed in disinfectant or forced to eat their own vomit. One girl had been made to clear a blocked toilet by removing the accumulated excrement with her bare hands.

On 14 January 2015, a statement from the Sisters of Nazareth accepted that children in their care had been abused. They offered their sincere and unreserved apology to all those whom they failed to protect.[26] A similar apology was made by the De La Salle Brothers on 11 December 2014.[27] At the session on 11 February 2015, the Sisters of Nazareth also expressed their 'sincere apologies and deep sadness at the pain and distress suffered by so many men and women as a result of the Child Migration Scheme'.[28]

In January 2017, the inquiry's report found that nuns had physically and emotionally abused children in their care, and that many incidents relating to sexual abuse were known by members of the clergy who did nothing to stop them. It recommended that victims should receive compensation, a public apology and a memorial.

Independent Inquiry into Child Sexual Abuse

On 7 July 2014, the Independent Inquiry into Child Sexual Abuse (IICSA) in England and Wales was announced by the Home Secretary, Theresa May. The first two individuals appointed to chair the Inquiry, Baroness Butler-Sloss and Fiona Woolf, both stepped down after accusations by abuse victims that they could not be impartial, due to various personal connections. In February 2015, IICSA was given the status of a 'statutory' inquiry, giving it powers to require sworn testimony and to have access to classified information. At around the same time, a New Zealand High Court judge, Dame Lowell Goddard QC, was appointed chair of the inquiry panel.

The inquiry opened on 9 July 2015. The first phase of work was to include twelve areas of investigation:

1. Children in the Care of Lambeth Council
2. Children in the Care of Nottinghamshire Councils
3. Cambridge House, Knowl View and Rochdale Council
4. Child Sexual Abuse in the Anglican Church
5. Child Sexual Abuse in the Roman Catholic Church
6. The Sexual Abuse of Children in Custodial Institutions
7. Child Sexual Abuse in Residential Schools
8. The Internet and Child Sexual Abuse
9. Child Exploitation by Organized Networks
10. The Protection of Children Outside the United Kingdom
11. Accountability and Reparations for Victims and Survivors
12. Allegations of Child Sexual Abuse Linked to Westminster[29]

In May 2016, it was reported that police were expecting to receive as many as 30,000 new child abuse reports by the time the Goddard Inquiry had concluded.[30]

A further change of chair came in August 2016 after Justice Goddard announced her resignation from the role, citing the difficulty of relinquishing her professional and family ties in New Zealand, and the 'legacy of failure' that the inquiry had acquired. She also warned that the inquiry was 'too big, unwieldy and under-funded to succeed'.[31] On 11 August 2016, it was announced that the inquiry would now be headed by Professor Alexis Jay, an existing member of its panel. The inquiry was now due to begin its hearings in March 2017. Another setback came on 30 September 2016, with the resignation of the inquiry's most senior lawyer, Ben Emmerson QC.

Scottish Child Abuse Inquiry

The Scottish Child Abuse Inquiry was established in 2015 to investigate the nature and extent of historic child abuse in Scotland covering the period which is within living memory of any person who suffered such abuse. Susan O'Brien QC was appointed as chair but resigned in July 2016, following claims that she had made 'unacceptable' comments relating to a child abuse victim.[32] She was succeeded by the Right Honourable Lady Anne Smith.

Kendall House, Gravesend

In 2016, an independent review took place concerning claims of abuse between the 1960s and 1980s at the Kendall House Home in Gravesend, run by the Church of England. The home, which closed in 1986, accommodated girls aged from 11 to 16 who often had serious behavioural or emotional problems. The review's findings[33] were described by its authors as 'harrowing'. Girls as young as 11 were routinely given high levels of sedatives and other drugs to control their behaviour, placing them in a constant stupor. As well as suffering from serious side-effects, the drugs made them vulnerable to emotional, physical and sexual abuse. Girls who tried to resist the drugs were often isolated in a locked room for long periods, or injected with powerful sedatives. Straitjackets were also sometimes used. Two former inmates alleged that they had been raped while in the isolation room. The report made nineteen recommendations for the diocesan authorities to address.

After releasing the report, the Bishop of Rochester, the Right Reverend James Langstaff, said he was 'appalled and saddened' by what he had learned and 'truly sorry that former residents were hurt and damaged by the actions of people at Kendall House who should have been providing them with a nurturing environment, care and support'.[34]

Legislative Changes

Abuse inquiries have invariably concluded with recommendations for lessons to be learned and changes in the policies, procedures or culture of the organizations involved, such as a far greater willingness for the allegations of victims to be taken seriously by officials and the police.

The increasing concern about the abuse of children in care has also been reflected in more recent legislation. The Criminal Records Bureau (CRB), which began operation in 2002, allowed employers to check on the backgrounds of individuals whose work would bring them into contact with children. In 2013, the CRB was replaced by the Disclosure and Barring Service, whose checks include more rigorous police screening.

Of wider significance was the 2004 Children Act which required local authorities to appoint a Director of Children's Services, to promote co-operation between agencies, and to set up Local Safeguarding Children's Boards. Other measures included the creation of a Children's Commissioner for England, and for guidance to be given regarding the setting up of databases holding basic information about children and young people to help professionals work together to provide early support to children, young people and their families.

Whether these changes will finally put an end to the shocking catalogue of abuse that has been suffered by children in care still remains to be seen.

Chapter 23

A Future for Children's Homes?

A study in 1998 presented a rather depressing view of the then state of children's residential care.[1] The homes often suffered from neglect by their local authorities, standards of care were uneven, and the majority of the establishments examined had not produced the written Statement of Purpose required by the Department of Health regulations[2] to spell out their aims, objectives and working practices. There were also generally poor relationships between social services departments and other children's agencies, such as psychology services or schools. The researchers were particularly struck by the fact that of the twenty homes they had looked at in a similar study ten years earlier, only four were now still in operation.

In recent decades, the use of children's residential care has fallen dramatically. At its peak in the mid-1970s, local authorities housed about 40,000 children – approximately 40 per cent of all those in their care. At the end of March 2015, the number being accommodated had fallen to 8,320, around 12 per cent of the national total of what are now referred to as 'looked after children'. Of those being housed, 5,290 (64 per cent) lived in children's homes, 180 were in secure accommodation, 1,100 lived in hostels (generally as part of moving out of care) and 670 were placed in residential schools.[3] The annual cost of caring for those living in children's homes was around £750 million, with the average cost of provision running at around £2,900 per child per week.[4] Of the 1,795 children's homes operating in 2015, about 21 per cent were run by local authorities, 6 per cent by the voluntary sector, and 73 per cent by commercial providers. Most placements were now short term, with 35 per cent lasting less than a month, and 82 per cent less than a year.[5]

The Narey Report

The declining use of residential care, its poor image, its high cost, the growing dominance of commercial providers, and the apparently endless number cases of abuse suffered by children living in the homes, raise a number of questions about its future. Are children's homes still relevant or are they now a relic of a bygone age? Do they provide value for money or are exorbitant profits being made by the businesses that now run most of them? Can the homes be made safe for the children that live in them? And are there any better solutions? These are the kinds of issues that, in October 2015, Sir Martin Narey was commissioned to investigate in an independent review of children's residential care in England. His report,[6] published in July 2016, provides an interesting snapshot of current residential provision, how it is run, and the characteristics of those placed in it.

Narey noted that the profile of those now being placed in children's homes is rather different to what it was in the past. The children are older on average, with three-quarters aged between 14 and 17, and the majority (62 per cent) being male. The children who live in homes have high levels of behavioural and emotional difficulties, with more than half of them having special educational needs. Research in 2013 found that 62 per cent of those in homes had clinically significant mental health problems, and 74 per cent had been violent or aggressive in the past six months. The most common reason for a child being placed in a home is their abuse or neglect, followed by family dysfunction.[7]

Despite the challenges placed by such children, the 2015 report by Ofsted, the government's inspection and regulation body, rated almost three-quarters of children's homes as 'good' or 'outstanding', and only 1 per cent as 'inadequate'.[8] In recognizing the vital contribution of the children's home workforce to this success, Narey was keen that undue importance should not be placed on their formal qualifications, or lack of them. The best staff, he suggested, were those with the vital ability to make and maintain good relationships with children who are troubled and challenging, and sometimes hard to like. As one care leaver had put it to him:

> *Staff in residential care simply need to be caring and this does not require a degree. They need some knowledge and training but a mixed skill set worked. The home formed its own family. There would be staff I would talk to about my problems, staff I would talk with if I wanted to laugh, and staff I would talk to if I wanted advice on clothes or make up. It worked wonderfully for me.[9]*

Narey recommended that the Department for Education should identify best practice in recruitment of staff to children's homes. This included screening out those who might not be up to the immense challenge presented by the work. In addition, providers should promote continuing staff development, particularly through team-based training. As many social work students as possible should spend part of their placement experience in children's homes.

A New Style of Home

Since 1946, when the Curtis Committee made its influential report, fostering has been seen as preferable, wherever possible, to placement in a children's home. Other factors aside, it is a much cheaper option – at the present time, the weekly cost of foster care for each child is about £600, while a place in a children's home is almost five times that amount.[10] However, there are some children, adolescents in particular, who determinedly resist fostering and for whom residential care may provide a better and more stable alternative to a succession of failed foster placements.

A contrary view, that a family placement is ultimately the best option for every child, has been pursued by the much-praised No Wrong Door (NWD) project run by North Yorkshire County Council. The scheme revolves around two 'hubs', located in Harrogate and Scarborough, which have replaced the council's traditional children's homes with a co-ordinated range of integrated provision for those in care and those leaving care. The facilities provided by the hubs include residential care home beds, emergency residential beds, community foster family placements, supported accommodation, and supported lodgings and outreach support. Each hub has a multi-disciplinary team which includes social workers and health professionals, including specialists such as a communications therapist and life coach. There is also a supportive police role. A core principle of the NWD scheme is that each young person it deals with has one key worker who works with him or her throughout their time in care. The NWD model also aims to blur the gap between foster and residential care, with prospective foster carers spending time working in a residential home to get to know a child they might eventually care for. Wherever possible, children moving to and fro between residential care and foster placements keep the same foster carers. As well as appearing to achieve better outcomes for children, the NWD scheme is proving financially attractive, with annual savings of up to £90,000 being achieved for each child.[11]

The Costs of Residential Care

The finances of providing children's residential care are complex. Although around a quarter of the commercially operated homes are run by just eleven private companies, the majority of providers

(71 per cent) have just one or two homes.[12] Most local authorities participate in regional purchasing consortia, but they deal with providers in a variety of different ways. These include individually contracting with providers chosen from an approved list, framework agreements for the purchase of specified services at agreed prices, the block purchase of beds from one or more providers, and cost-and-volume contracts where prices are reduced as the authority's spend increases. Narey concluded that local authorities needed to do much better at exploiting their purchasing power and make more use of block contract arrangements. The latter, which typically offer providers a much higher occupancy rate for their places, can result in them being able to offer lower prices.[13]

Narey also suggested that authorities make more use of schemes such as Link Maker[14] which provide information on the availability of places with different providers. The use of such resources might also benefit those children placed in homes away from their own communities. In 2015, around 63 per cent of children in foster care resided within their own local authority area, while for those in residential homes the figure was only 41 per cent. Of those placed in homes further afield, most were placed at a distance of between fifty and 100 miles, but some were more than 150 miles away, the furthest being 271 miles.[15] There are sometimes, however, positive reasons for distant placements such as to access specialist provision for children with complex disabilities or severe mental health issues, or to use geographical distance to help break patterns of risky behaviour such as involvement in gangs or sexual exploitation.[16]

Despite occasional suggestions of excessive profit-making by the private sector, the average weekly cost of places from private suppliers is virtually the same as that in homes run by local authorities themselves. Given that the charges made by private providers must include an element of profit, the obvious conclusion is that local authority homes are not being run as efficiently as they might be. Nary reported that staffing levels are generally lower in privately run homes and some deploy their staff in more effective ways, for example in having fewer staff on duty during daytime hours when their residents are usually out.[17] The general move to smaller accommodation units, with four beds now being the average, is also making places more expensive. There appears to be little evidence to suggest that homes of this size are any more beneficial to their residents than those with eight or ten places.[18]

Another of Narey's suggestions was that encouragement could be given to the voluntary sector to increase its contribution to the market.

He recognized, however, that large charities such as Barnardo's, which once dominated this work, had been scarred by memories of the numerous historic child abuse scandals.[19]

Managing Inmates

An issue that has received much public attention in recent years is how the staff at children's homes deal with particularly difficult behaviour, particularly that coming into the category of criminal acts, such as physical violence or damage to property. A particular concern is the involvement of the police in such cases, with the result that a child might be criminalized for some apparently minor misdemeanour that should have been sorted out by the home itself. Maintaining order and discipline in a children's home can clearly be a challenge although a very long way removed far from the impression sometimes given by the media.

Much prominence was given to a 2015 report produced by the Howard League which found that over a twelve-month period, the Sussex police had received at total of 3,500 call-outs from the forty-seven children's homes in the county. In fact, less than 10 per cent of these related to criminal activity, while most related the safety and welfare of children leaving the home. Increasingly, even in cases of serious assault or damage to property, the managers of homes avoid involving the police, except to calm a situation. Instead, there is a growing use of restorative justice approaches where face-to-face meetings and group work allow victims to be heard and for offenders to have the opportunity of accepting responsibility for their actions.[20]

One area of confusion among some residential care staff has concerned what powers they have in forcibly confining a child. One specific recommendation made by the Narey Report on this matter was for the Department for Education 'to ensure that staff are able to keep children safe by preventing them leaving homes at time of danger, either by locking doors or using restraint, and that they can be confident in the legality of their doing so'.[21]

Staying Put?

The transition from care into independent adult life has always been viewed as a time when young people are in particular need of support. In 2013, the government announced the introduction of an arrangement known as 'Staying Put', to allow children in foster care to remain with their foster families after reaching the age of eighteen. Although widely welcomed, the scheme was also criticized as not being extended to include those in children's homes. The difficulties of doing so would be considerable, however. Apart from the financial costs, the continuing presence of young adults in a children's home might raise concerns about a variety of safeguarding issues such as their use of alcohol and drugs, partying, arguing with staff etc.

An alternative proposal, 'Staying Close' rather than 'Staying Put', where leavers could live in their own flat located very close to their former children's home, might allow them to retain the close contact but avoid many of the problems, and also be a much cheaper option. There have also been moves to enable local authorities to offer support to those leaving children's homes through the provision of a personal adviser to each care leaver.[22]

Looking to the Future

Although the Narey Report was very clear that children's homes could be improved, its author was ultimately optimistic about their future:

> [T]he role of children's homes is misunderstood, the challenge of the children they care for underestimated, and the contribution they make too easily dismissed. Three-quarters of homes are good or better. Some are genuinely outstanding. I have been moved by some of what I've seen. What they can achieve, is captured brilliantly here by one care leaver, who looks back on her experience with gratitude and affection: 'Residential care was my home, it was my life and it is still a big memory ... Residential care absolutely turned my life around and I now am in a position where I am studying social work and giving back to the community ... This would not have happened should I have remained in foster care.'[23]

Chapter 24

Children's Home Records

Locating any surviving historical records for a particular children's establishment can often prove difficult and frustrating. A large number of homes were privately operated and it is often the case that the groups that once ran them no longer exist. Over the years, some homes changed their management, their location or their name. Even for those that were run by statutory bodies such as boards of guardians or local councils, there was until relatively recently no formal obligation to preserve records relating to those in their care. Even when the storage of records was undertaken, events over the years such as fire, flood, and wartime destruction might have taken their toll.

Getting Started

If you are trying to locate records for yourself, or for someone you know (or suspect) was in some kind of children's home, a good first step is to organize and write down all the information you already know or can obtain first-hand. If the person is an ancestor in the more distant past, then it is worth spending the time to do some initial groundwork.

Family memories are always useful to record, even if fairly vague, but remember that the circumstances that led to a child ending up in institutional care, such as poverty, illegitimacy or marital break-up, were often considered shameful. You may find that people are reluctant to talk about details or were themselves told a false or misleading story to cover up embarrassing events, such as a workhouse being referred to as an 'orphanage'. Considerable sensitivity may therefore be required when exploring such matters.

Other family material in the form of letters, photos, and newspaper cuttings may also prove useful in your research. People often find it difficult to pinpoint exact dates, but can often give relative dates, e.g. 'it was just before the war started', or 'it was the year after Auntie Mary died' which can indirectly help place events.

The ideal starting point is the birth certificate for the person concerned – their birth date, full name, mother's name etc. may help confirm that an inmate recorded at a home is definitely the person you're looking for.

Having a census record for the person while they were in the institution will also be a great help. Civil registration indexes and census records are available online via a number of commercial sources including:

- Ancestry (www.ancestry.co.uk)
- Findmypast (www.findmypast.co.uk)
- Genes Reunited (www.genesreunited.co.uk)
- The Genealogist (www.thegenealogist.co.uk)

The Free UK Genealogy project (www.freeukgenealogy.org.uk) includes transcriptions of census records and birth/death registration indexes. Although free to use, it is not yet complete in its coverage. Also free is the UKBMD website (www.ukbmd.org.uk) which provides links to other sites holding census transcriptions or indexes – this includes local register offices that provide online index searching.

Identifying the Institution

Identifying the particular institution (or institutions) where a child once resided can sometimes be tricky. Family memories can be notoriously unreliable when it comes to exact names and locations. Larger towns and cities sometimes had several children's homes whose names could easily be confused. This is not helped by the fact that, over the years, some institutions were renamed or relocated.

Often you may at least know the county or town where the home was located. If you first encounter a home via a census listing, its identity may not be immediately clear as the names given to institutions by census enumerators can sometimes be rather terse or cryptic. My website www.childrenshomes.org.uk can help you browse the details of homes in a particular area, and also gives detailed information on many hundreds of individual establishments. Alternatively, consulting old trade directories for the area may help you pinpoint the home in question. The 'Trades Directory' section at the back of many Kelly's directories usually includes a 'Homes' section listing the various institutional homes operating in the area at a particular date. A large online collection of trade directories from England and Wales is available free in the Historical Directories collection (specialcollections.le.ac.uk/cdm), while commercial sites such as Ancestry (www.ancestry.co.uk) are increasingly adding trade directories to their resources.

Old Ordnance Survey maps often identify larger orphanages and children's homes, with websites such as www.old-maps.co.uk and maps.nls.uk/os being useful online resources for this purpose.

If the home was run by an organization such as Dr Barnardo's, an occupational body, or was a Reformatory or Industrial School, this should be apparent from its name or other details. Homes run by boards of guardians – the local workhouse authority in each Poor Law union area – usually include the word 'Union' or 'Guardians' in their descriptions.

General Search Resources

Some useful resources that you may find helpful in locating children's home records are:

- www.childrenshomes.org.uk – see the records available for hundreds of children's institutions
- discovery.nationalarchives.gov.uk – search the catalogues of over 2,500 local archives in England and Wales
- archiveshub.ac.uk – search the catalogues of over 300 specialist UK archives
- When using the search facility on each of these websites, be prepared to try different combinations of the name and location of the home you're looking for, e.g. liverpool girls orphanage, newcastle nazareth house, bedfordshire children's home

Access to Records

Regardless of the type of institution you are researching, there may well be access restrictions on viewing its records. To comply with current data protection legislation, most record repositories do not allow the viewing of material containing personal information for a period of up to 100 years from the date of the latest entry in a particular volume. In the case of more recent records, however, archives may be able to provide individuals with information about themselves, subject to proof of identity being supplied.

Poor Law Children's Homes

From the 1840s onwards, boards of guardians increasingly provided separate accommodation for children away from their union workhouses. A number of different types of establishment were gradually developed including district schools, cottage homes, and scattered homes.

As well as the homes they ran themselves, boards of guardians also placed children in accommodation run by others. Many were boarded out (fostered) with individual families. Some, especially Roman Catholics and children with special needs, were sent to Certified Schools.

Before being placed in one of the various types of home, children entering the poor relief system usually spent an initial period in a workhouse or central home and would appear in its admission records. The individual homes also kept their own separate admission, discharge and other registers.

Surviving union records are now usually located in the relevant county or metropolitan record office for the area – www.workhouses.org.uk has details of location and extent of records that exist for each union.

The Ancestry website (www.ancestry.co.uk) has a large collection of London admission workhouse records, and some from unions in Dorset, Norfolk, Warwickshire, West Yorkshire and Medway in Kent. The Findmypast website (www.findmypast.co.uk) has a variety of workhouse records from Westminster, Cheshire, Derbyshire, Lincolnshire, the Manchester area, Monmouthshire and Dublin. With both these websites, a subscription is required for full access.

Local Authority Children's Homes

In 1930, the boards of guardians that ran the workhouse system were abolished and the administration of the poor relief system passed to county and county borough councils. This included the operation of homes for pauper children. Surviving records for the homes from this period are often to be found in the same record offices as those of their predecessor unions.

Following the 1948 Children Act, local authorities established Children's Departments to run the education and welfare services for children in their area. In 1971, Children's Departments and their functions were absorbed into new Social Services departments.

Prior to 1991, there was no legal requirement for councils to retain the records of children leaving their care, and the survival of all such records is very variable. Older records may sometimes now have been placed with the relevant county, city or borough record office. Many of these offices now have online catalogues of their holdings and also contribute to the National Archives' Discovery facility (discovery. nationalarchives.gov.uk).

More recent records for council-run children's homes are most likely to be held in each council's own internal archives. A list of the local authority contact details for enquiries is provided on the website of the

Care Leavers Association (www.careleavers.com/accesstorecords/ database). The website also gives guidance and advice on accessing childhood care files, which are usually only open to the individuals they relate to.

Some files relating to council-run homes, for example inspection reports, though not inmate registers, are held by the UK National Archives.

Charity Organizations

Many children's homes were run by national or local charities. Some of these are still in existence, although often having undergone one or more changes of name over the years, for example the former National Children's Home is now Action for Children. A number of these organizations operate well-organized enquiry services relating to their records. Access to case records may incur a charge and be restricted to requests from former inmates or, in the case of individuals now deceased, their immediate descendants (subject to proof of death being provided). A counselling service may also be offered for those accessing their own records. Some charities, such as Barnardo's, have handed their administrative records over to another body, such as a public archive or academic library, but retained their children's personal case records.

- **Barnardo's**
  Barnardo's (www.barnardos.org.uk) has a Family History service which deals with enquiries regarding records of individual children. Its Making Connections service is for those wishing to access their own Barnardo's adoption records. Barnardo's historical administrative records are now deposited with Liverpool University's Social Welfare Archives (www.liv.ac.uk/library/ sca/colldescs/social.html) with prior written permission needed from Barnardo's for access. Barnardo's also holds records for organizations it took over including the Liverpool Sheltering Homes, Macpherson Homes, Miss Sharman's Homes, the Reformatory and Refuge Union and the Children's Aid Society.

- **Action for Children (formerly National Children's Home)**
  Action for Children (www.actionforchildren.org.uk) provides access to care records for people who were adopted through the charity or who resided in one of its homes. Currently this service is only available to the individuals concerned and not to the descendants of deceased former residents.

- **The Children's Society (formerly Waifs and Strays)**
  The Children's Society (www.childrenssociety.org.uk) has a Post-Adoption and Care service (email: postadoption@childrenssociety.org.uk) which provides access to records, information, advice, birth record counselling, tracing and intermediary service for people who were in care or adopted through the Society. Files for children admitted to its homes after September 1926 were microfilmed in the 1980s and the originals destroyed. Some post-1926 files had already been damaged or destroyed by a flood. Detailed catalogues are available for its holdings relating to disabled children (www.hiddenlives.org.uk/including_the_excluded/completed_catalogues.html).

Similar arrangements may exist for other surviving organizations that still maintain their own archives.

Some charities have handed their records over to other repositories. For example, the records of Shaftesbury Young People (the former Shaftesbury Homes) are now at the London Metropolitan Archives (www.cityoflondon.gov.uk/lma). For institutions which, after their closure, evolved into charitable trusts, the Charity Commission website (www.gov.uk/government/organisations/charity-commission) may have contact details. For homes that were run by long-vanished organizations, try discovery.nationalarchives.gov.uk or the county/metropolitan record office covering the area.

Religious Organizations

Children's homes were operated by a number of religious groups and organizations. Records from the Church of England's Waifs and Strays Society and the Methodists' National Children's Home have already been referred to above. Other groups linked to the Church of England include:

- **The Girls' Friendly Society**
  The Society's archives are now at the Women's Library at the London School of Economics (twl-calm.library.lse.ac.uk/CalmView/record.aspx?src=CalmView.Catalog&id=5GFS). Records relating to some of its branches are held at local archives – try discovery.nationalarchives.gov.uk

- **The Ladies' Association for the Care of Friendless Girls**
  Records relating for a few branches are held at local archives – try discovery.nationalarchives.gov.uk

Many Roman Catholic children's homes were organized within Catholic diocesan areas and run by a branch of the Catholic Children's Society, perhaps in conjunction with a particular religious order. Where the (often now renamed) Children's Society or order is still active, it may hold records for the homes that they operated. Alternatively, records may have been placed in the relevant county or Catholic diocesan archives. The web page at www.childrenshomes.org.uk/research/ religious.shtml includes website or email contact details for a number of Catholic diocesan and childcare organizations, and for Catholic and Anglican religious orders that ran establishments for the care of children or young people.

Some of the Catholic orders that became involved in the running of children's homes have names that may prove perplexingly similar. For example, the Sisters of Charity of St Paul the Apostle, the Sisters of Charity of Jesus and Mary, the Sisters of Charity of Our Lady Mother of Mercy, the Irish Sisters of Charity, and the Daughters of Charity of St Vincent de Paul (not to be confused with the St Vincent de Paul Society) may all sometimes be referred to simply as the 'Sisters of Charity'. Likewise, the 'Christian Brothers' may denote either the Irish (Edmund Rice) Christian Brothers or De La Salle Brothers (Brothers of the Christian Schools).

Those researching Catholic ancestors in the UK may also be interested in the activities of the Catholic Family History Society (catholicfhs.co.uk/).

Reformatories, Industrial and Approved Schools

The reformatory system in England began in 1854, with Certified Industrial Schools following in 1857. The two types of institution were merged in 1933 and replaced by Approved Schools. The majority of these establishments were run by charitable or religious groups and the survival of their records is very uneven.

Most of those entering Reformatories and Industrial Schools were placed there by the courts and details of their committal proceedings recorded in local magistrates' (Petty Sessions) records. These are generally found in the county or metropolitan archives of the place where the sentencing took place – this may be some distance from the institution where the young person subsequently became an inmate. It should also be noted that many of these establishments also took voluntary admissions, whose details will not appear in court records.

A few of these institutions were run by the major charities including Barnardo's, the National Children's Home and the Waifs and Strays Society, whose details are noted above. A similar situation applies to institutions of this type run by other bodies (e.g. religious groups) which still survive and which maintain their own archives. Access to such records may incur a charge and also be restricted to former inmates or their immediate descendants.

Because they were subject to government inspection, many documents relating to the operation of these institutions are held at the National Archives. Otherwise, the best place to look for surviving records is the record office covering the area where a particular establishment was located.

Records for several Reformatories and Industrial Schools in West Yorkshire are now available online via Ancestry (ancestry.co.uk).

Other Homes

The survival of records for the large number of smaller independent children's homes is generally very limited and is more likely to feature administrative documents rather than details of inmates. A good place to start your search is with one of the websites listed in the General Search Resources section above. For example, a search on discovery. nationalarchives.gov.uk for 'Railway Servants Orphanage' indicates that admission and discharge registers for that institution are held in the Derbyshire Record Office.

The records for smaller institutions are most likely to have survived where the operators of such establishments still exist in some shape or form, such as Coram (coram.org.uk) who formerly ran London's Foundling Hospital.

A few children's home records may be found via commercial family history websites, for example findmypast.co.uk has the Derby Railway Servants' Orphanage registers (1875–1912) and ancestry.co.uk has lists of children at the Royal Female Orphanage, Beddington (1890–1913).

Adoption and Fostering Records

Prior to 1927, child adoption in England and Wales was arranged on an informal basis by many organizations including workhouse authorities and the operators of orphanages and other children's institutions. However, such placements gave the adoptive parents no legal rights. A child's biological parents could turn up at any time and demand it be returned to their custody. This situation was changed by the Adoption of Children Act of 1926 which introduced a legally regulated adoption system. Similar legislation was enacted in Scotland in 1930 and in Northern Ireland in 1931.

On 1 January 1927, a central Adopted Children Register was created to record the basic details of all adoptions under the new system. Children adopted from this date can apply to find out their original birth record – see the UK government's Adoption Records web page (www.gov.uk/adoption-records) for details.

Another government-run service is the Adoption Contact Register (www.gov.uk/adoption-records/the-adoption-contact-register) which allows you to find a birth relative or an adopted person, or to say that you don't want to be contacted.

For any surviving records regarding the adoption process itself (possibly including pre-1927 'adoptions'), you will need to contact the organization or institution that arranged the adoption, or the successor body that inherited its records. A useful resource to help locate adoption records is the Adoption Search Reunion website (www.adoptionsearchreunion.org.uk/search/adoptionrecords).

Fostering (boarding out) records are most likely to be located with any other surviving children's records of the institution or organization concerned.

Emigration Records

As well as the records held by the various UK organizations that migrated children, a variety of other resources exist relating to many thousands of British Home Children who were migrated to countries such as Canada and Australia. These include records such as ship passenger lists, immigration forms, and official reports on follow-up visits to child immigrants. Much of this material is now available online and some useful websites are listed below:

- www.bac-lac.gc.ca/eng/discover/immigration – an extensive collection of information from Library and Archives Canada.
- canadianbritishhomechildren.weebly.com – British Home Children in Canada
- www.dcs.uwaterloo.ca/~marj/genealogy/homeadd.html – 'Young Immigrants to Canada' by Marj Kohli
- personal.uwaterloo.ca/marj/genealogy/children/tracers.html– sources of help in tracing emigrants by Marj Kohli
- guides.naa.gov.au/good-british-stock – a research guide on child and youth migration to Australia by Barry Coldrey

The National Archives

The UK National Archives (TNA), based at Kew, holds a large number of records relating to children's residential care institutions. However, these are largely concerned with administrative and policy matters rather than the inmates and staff of these establishments. A research guide about the TNA's holdings on children's homes is available at: www.nationalarchives.gov.uk/help-with-your-research/research-guides/children-care

Records at the TNA for individual institutions include:

- Inspection reports – from 1933, all children's homes funded by voluntary contributions were subject to Home Office inspection. This was extended to all other homes from 1948. TNA holds copies of these reports, which appraise each establishment's premises, staff, operation etc.
- Inquiries – the results of special investigations into complaints or other incidents.
- Correspondence – between government departments and institutions on administrative matters.
- The TNA also holds more general material such as statistical returns and reports, copies of circulars, instructions and other documents issued to local authorities and institutions, and correspondence between government departments and other bodies such as charities, committees of inquiry etc.

A growing number of National Archives records are now viewable online free, while copies of other documents can be ordered on payment of a fee.

Chapter 25

Useful Resources

Websites

www.childrenshomes.org.uk – information on many thousands of children's institutions and the organizations that ran them.

www.workhouses.org.uk – details of many of the individual children's institutions operated by the Poor Law authorities.

www.barnardos.org.uk/what_we_do/our_history.htm – a history of Barnardo's including a directory of its former homes.

www.hiddenlives.org.uk – a rich archive of material from the Children's Society (formerly Waifs and Strays) including the Society's homes, publications and sample case files.

www.theirhistory.co.uk – an extensive collection of historical material about the National Children's Home compiled by former inmate Philip Howard.

www.youtube.com – has historical items featuring children's homes, especially Barnardo's and National Children's Home, many from Movietone and British Pathé archives. Some vintage NCH films can be found on the channel 'philipastrangechild'.

www.coram.org.uk/about-us/our-heritage-foundling-hospital – the story of Thomas Coram and the Foundling Hospital.

leicester.contentdm.oclc.org/cdm/landingpage/collection/p16445coll4 – historical directories of England and Wales.

maps.nls.uk – historical Ordnance Survey maps of Great Britain.

www.britishnewspaperarchive.co.uk – a massive archive of local and regional newspapers (subscription required).

newspapers.library.wales – Welsh newspapers online.

www.thetcj.org – *Therapeutic Care Journal* (formerly *Children Webmag*). Has a rich archive of useful articles, notably its Key Texts series.

www.cchn.org.uk – the Child Care History Network.

www.connectedhistories.org – a facility to search multiple online historical sources (1500–1900).

www.gov.uk/government/publications/childrens-homes-data-pack – current statistics on children's home provision.

www.iicsa.org.uk – the Independent Inquiry into Child Sexual Abuse.

www.childabusecommission.ie – the Irish Child Abuse Commission.

www.hiainquiry.org – the Northern Ireland Historical Institutional Abuse Inquiry.

www.childabuseinquiry.scot – the Scottish Child Abuse Inquiry.

Places to Visit

foundlingmuseum.org.uk – the Foundling Hospital Museum, London.

www.mullers.org/heritage – the Müller Museum, Bristol.

www.bristolmuseums.org.uk/red-lodge-museum – the Red Lodge Museum, Bristol.

riponmuseums.co.uk/museums/workhouse_museum_gardens – Ripon Workhouse Museum.

www.museums.norfolk.gov.uk/visit_us/gressenhall_farm_and_workhouse – Gressenhall Farm and Workhouse, Norfolk.

weaverhall.westcheshiremuseums.co.uk – Weaver Hall Museum and Workhouse, Northwich.

www.nationaltrust.org.uk/the-workhouse-southwell – The Workhouse, Southwell.

www.nationaltrust.org.uk/quarry-bank – Quarry Bank Mill, Styal, Cheshire.

www.raggedschoolmuseum.org.uk – the Ragged School Museum, London.

References and Notes

Note: References to British Parliamentary Papers are prefaced by 'PP' with the paper number, where applicable, included in brackets.

Chapter 1: Early Children's Homes

1. Manzione, 1995, pp. 35-36
2. Lawson and Silver, 1973, p. 202
3. McConville, 1981, p. 32
4. Leonard, 1900, pp. 354-355
5. Pearl, 1978, p. 226
6. Strype, 1720, p. 199
7. Lawson and Silver, 1973, p. 182
8. Trimmer, 1792, p. 12
9. *Victoria County History of York*, p. 91
10. Jones M. G., 1938, p. 103
11. Nichols and Wray, 1935, p. 31
12. *Ibid.*, p.58
13. Hughson, 1807, p. 533
14. Partington, 1834, p. 43
15. *Ibid.*
16. PP *Digest of Schools and Charities for Education*, 1843 (435) – 'Schools Not Classical' section.

Chapter 2: Reformatories, Ragged and Industrial Schools

1. Barnett, 1913, p. 17
2. *Ibid.*
3. Russell, 1906, p. 205
4. Dickens, 1851, p. 547
5. Guthrie, 1849, p. 76
6. *Bristol Mercury*, 26 December 1846, p. 4
7. *Ibid.*
8. *The Fireside Annual*, 1880, p. 562
9. *Evening Mail*, London, 12 May, 1852, p. 8
10. PP *Annual Reports of Inspector of Reformatory and Industrial Schools*
11. PP *Thirty-fifth Report of Inspector of Reformatory and Industrial Schools*, 1892 (C. 6733), p. 222

12. PP *Thirty-eighth Report of Inspector of Reformatory and Industrial Schools,* 1895 (C. 7820), p. 228
13. Gloucestershire Archives D3549/25/3/9
14. Havers, 2006
15. PP *Forty-second Report of Inspector of Reformatory and Industrial Schools,* 1899 (C. 9450), p. 192
16. PP *General Rules for the Management and Discipline of Certified Industrial Schools,* 1893–4 (C. 7118), p. 5
17. National Archives, HO 45/14545
18. PP *Third Report of Inspector of Reformatory Schools,* 1860 (2668), p. 40
19. PP *Report of Departmental Committee on Reformatory and Industrial Schools,* 1913 (Cd. 6838), p. 7
20. PP *Report of Departmental Committee on Treatment of Young Offenders,* 1927 (Cmd. 2831), p. 72

Chapter 3: Approved Schools

1. Hyland, 1993, p. 21
2. Parker, 1990, p. 51
3. Home Office, 1951, p. 64
4. Kirkwood, 1992, p. 11
5. Advisory Council on Child Care, 1970, p. 4
6. Hyland, 1993, p. 117

Chapter 4: Training Ships

1. Carradice, 2009, p. 63

Chapter 5: The Shaftesbury Homes and 'Arethusa'

1. Kohli, William John Pady, 2016, pp. 14-15
2. *London Evening Standard,* 15 February 1866, p. 3
3. *Liverpool Mercury,* 11 July 1868, p. 5
4. Anonymous (n.d.)
5. Bailey, 1996, p. 137
6. *Ibid.,* p. 138
7. *Ibid.,* p. 145

Chapter 6: Müller's Orphan Houses

1. Tayler, 1871, pp. 55-56
2. *Ibid.,* p. 181 (Abridged)

Chapter 7: Barnardo's Homes

1. Wagner, 1979, p. 42
2. Charity Organisation Society, 1890, p. 295

3. Barnardo and Merchant, 1907, p. 156
4. Rose, 1987, p. 113
5. *Ibid.*, p. 185
6. www.childrenshomes.org.uk/DB/rules.shtml Retrieved 10 June 2016

Chapter 8: The National Children's Home

1. Bradfield, 1913, p. 78
2. Barritt, 1972, p. 14
3. Bradfield, 1913, p. 172
4. *Ibid.*, p.182
5. *Ibid.*, pp. 141-144
6. Jacka, 1969, p. 27
7. Philpot, 1994, pp. 43-44
8. *Ibid.*, pp. 44-45

Chapter 9: The Waifs and Strays Society

1. Stroud, 1971
2. *Ibid.*, p.25
3. *Ibid.*, pp. 43-44
4. *Ibid.*, p. 45
5. *Ibid.*, p. 51
6. *Ibid.*, p. 52
7. *Ibid.*, pp. 81-82
8. *Ibid.*, p. 83
9. *Ibid.*, p. 193
10. *Ibid.*, p.215
11. *Ibid.*, p. 218
12. *Ibid.*, p. 230

Chapter 10: Occupational Homes

1. Charity Organisation Society, 1890, p. 308
2. *Ibid.*, p. 323
3. *Ibid.*, p. 329
4. Ashby, 2013

Chapter 11: Other Voluntary Homes

1. Fullerton, 1930, p. 59
2. e.g. *Preston Chronicle*, 23 September 1893, p. 7
3. *Sevenoaks Chronicle and Kentish Advertiser*, 2 July 1920, p. 9
4. Charity Organisation Society, 1890, p. 339
5. Ray, 1903, p. 349

6. Charity Organisation Society, 1890, p. 312
7. Children's Aid Society, 50th Report, 1906, pp. 4-5

Chapter 12: Religious Homes

1. Charity Organisation Society, 1890, p. 323
2. Sisters of Nazareth, 2016
3. Gray-Wilson, 2000, pp. 38-40
4. Pinches, 1998, p. 29
5. Sandall, Wiggins, and Coutts, 1955, p. 157
6. Charity Organisation Society, 1890, p. 333
7. *Ibid.*, p. 241
8. *Ibid.*, p. 332

Chapter 13: Children with Disabilities

1. Smithers, 1825, p. 241
2. Anonymous, 1818, pp. 6-8
3. Charity Organisation Society, 1890, p. 34
4. *Ibid.*, p. 32
5. Philpott, 1904, p. 244
6. Gillard, 2011
7. Charity Organisation Society, 1890, pp. 25-65
8. Charity Organisation Society, 1893, pp. 119-120
9. Charity Organisation Society, 1890, p. 65
10. Ayers, 1971, p. 206
11. Gilbert, 1872, p. 277
12. Barnardo and Merchant, 1907, p. 130
13. Philpott, 1904, p. 278
14. Jones, 1972, p. 214
15. Oswin, 1975, pp. 71-72
16. Stoke Park Hospital – the Latter Years
17. PP *Royal Commission on Care and Control of the Feeble-Minded*, volume VIII, 1908 (Cd. 4202), p. 315
18. *Ibid.*, p. 316
19. *Ibid.*
20. Richardson, 1998, p. 110
21. *Ibid.*

Chapter 14: Fund Raising

1. Fletcher, 2005, pp. 111-112
2. *Ibid.*
3. Walpole, 1941, p. 177
4. Rudolf, 1922, p. 73
5. Barnardo and Merchant, 1907, p. 250

6. Founder's Day Programme, 1935 (An expenditure of £50,000 a year for the 8,000 or so children then in the charity's care equates to around 4d. per child per day.)
7. *Broken Wings* is viewable at www.youtube.com/watch?v=laQ9m71Xngg

Chapter 15: Poor Law Homes

1. Higginbotham, 2012, p. 298
2. Higginbotham, 2008, pp. 53-55
3. http://workhouses.org.uk/gco/gco1847.shtml (Articles 136–142) Retrieved 10 June 2016
4. PP *Appendix to Sixth Annual Report of Poor Law Commissioners*, 1840 (253), p. 135
5. Crompton, 1997, p. 154
6. PP *Fifth Annual Report of the Poor Law Commissioners*, 1839 (239), p. 99.
7. *Ibid.*, p. 99
8. Chaplin, 1979, pp. 22-23
9. The wife of Nassau John Senior and thus usually referred to at that time as Mrs Nassau Senior.
10. PP *Third Annual Report of Local Government Board*, 1874 (C. 1071), p. 341
11. *Proceedings of the Central and District Poor Law Conferences May 1904 to February 1905*, p. 38
12. PP *Fifth Annual Report of the Irish Poor Law Commissioners*, 1852 (1530), pp. 204-206
13. PP *Persons in Receipt of Poor-Law Relief*, 1922 (172), pp. 21-26
14. Hansard, 26 July 1922 vol. 157 col. 446

Chapter 16: Emigration Homes

1. Barnardo and Merchant, 1907, p. 164
2. Wagner, 1982, p. xv
3. Rye, 1870
4. PP *Pauper Children (Canada)*,1875 (9)
5. *Kelly's Directory of Liverpool and Suburbs*, 1894, p. 21 (abridged)
6. Parker, 2010, p. 192

Chapter 17: Boarding Out / Fostering

1. Barnardo and Merchant, 1907, p. 185
2. *An Act for the Better Relief and Employment of the Poor* 22 Geo. III, c. 83
3. PP *Copies of Report of J.J. Henley, Poor Law Inspector, to Poor Law Board, on Boarding out of Pauper Children*, 1870 (176), p. 36
4. Glen, 1879, pp. 444-453
5. Pinchbeck and Hewitt, 1973, p. 533

6. Stroud, 1971, p. 67
7. *Ibid.,* p. 70
8. Jacka, 1969, p. 27

Chapter 18: Aftercare and Preventive Work

1. PP *Fortieth Annual Report of Inspector of Reformatory and Industrial Schools,* 1897 (C.8566), p. 367
2. Charity Organisation Society, 1890, p. 281
3. *Ibid.,* p. 287
4. PP *Twenty-third Annual Report of Local Government Board,* 1894 (C. 7500), p. lxxxviii
5. Oldfield, 2008, p. 259
6. *Ibid.,* p. 261
7. http://girlsfriendlysociety.org.uk/history.html Retrieved 10 June 2016

Chapter 19: Magdalen Homes

1. Mahood, 1990, p. 78
2. Bartley, 2000, p. 48
3. Maddison, 1898, p. 214
4. *Ibid.,* p. 60
5. Pearce, 1958, p. 51
6. Charity Organisation Society, 1890, p. 527
7. Nokes, 1886, pp. 24-25
8. *Ibid.,* 19-20
9. Reformatory and Refuge Union, 1912, pp. 100-127
10. Charity Organisation Society, 1890, p. 528
11. Charity Organisation Society, 1939, p. 343
12. Reformatory and Refuge Union, 1912, p. 97

Chapter 20: Local Authority Children's Homes

1. Parker, 2015, p. 42
2. *Ibid.,* p. 44
3. Women's Group on Public Welfare, 1943, p. vii
4. Care of Children Committee, 1946, p. 2
5. *Ibid.,* pp. 39-40
6. *Ibid.,* p. 38
7. *Ibid.,* p. 72
8. *Ibid.,* p.75
9. *Ibid.*
10. *Ibid.,* p. 135
11. *Ibid.,* p. 179
12. Scottish Home Department, 1946, p. 15
13. Parker, 2015, pp. 70-74

14. Birmingham City Council Children's Department, 1953, p. 80
15. City of Manchester Children's Committee, 1956, pp. 48-49
16. PP *Children in the Care of Local Authorities in England and Wales*, 1952-53 (Cmd. 8910) and successive editions.
17. Parker, 2015, pp. 50-51
18. Cliffe and Berridge, 1991, p. 4
19. www.gov.uk/government/publications/childrens-homes-data-pack Retrieved 10 June 2016

Chapter 21: Life in Children's Homes

1. *Our Waifs and Strays*, August 1892, p. 6
2. Hitchman, 1966, p. 140
3. Urey, 1985, p. 16
4. Stroud, 1971, p. 112
5. *Ibid.*
6. *Ibid.*, p. 113
7. *Ibid.*, p.42
8. Gray-Wilson, 2000, p. 66
9. Hamblin, 2010, p. 5
10. Birmingham City Council Children's Department, 1953, pp. 118-119
11. Gray-Wilson, 2000, pp. 66-67
12. Rose, 1987, p. 210
13. Hitchman, 1966, p. 141
14. Berridge and Brodie, 1998, p. 91

Chapter 22: Abuse in Children's Homes

1. Wythen Baxter, 1841, pp. 155-156
2. www.workhouses.org.uk/Hackney Retrieved 10 June 2016
3. Smart, 2000, p. 57
4. *Yorkshire Post*, 16 July 1955, p. 4
5. Cummings, 2008
6. www.bbc.co.uk/news/uk-england-hampshire-27794784   Retrieved   10 June 2016
7. Levy and Kahan, 1990, p. 167
8. Utting, 1991
9. Kirkwood, 1992, p. 18
10. *Ibid.*
11. Warner, 1992
12. Waterhouse, 1999, p. 30
13. *Ibid.*, p. 788
14. *Ibid.*, pp. 788-789
15. Jillings, 1996, p. 250
16. *Ibid.*

17. www.bbc.co.uk/news/uk-england-manchester-20337495 Retrieved 10 June 2016

18. www.whatdotheyknow.com/request/215076/response/562609/ attach/7/8886%20Redacted.pdf Retrieved 10 June 2016

19. www.telegraph.co.uk/news/uknews/crime/9678697/Sir-Cyril-Smith-sex-abuse-dossier-seized-by-MI5.html Retrieved 10 June 2016

20. Danczuk, 2014

21. www.childabusecommission.ie/rpt/pdfs/CICA-VOL2-02.PDF, p. 46 Retrieved 10 June 2016

22. *Ibid.*, p. 30

23. *Ibid.*, p. 54

24. Ryan, 2009

25. www.childabusecommission.ie/rpt/pdfs/CICA-VOL4-13.PDF.   p.1 Retrieved 10 June 2016

26. www.hiainquiry.org/index/module_4_sisters_of_nazareth_belfast/ m4_d86_transcript_red_opt.pdf, p. 98 Retrieved 10 June 2016

27. www.hiainquiry.org/index/module_3_de_la_salle_boys_home_ at_rubane_house_kircubbin/m3_d78_transcript_red_opt.pdf, p. 11 Retrieved 10 June 2016

28. www.hiainquiry.org/index/module_4_sisters_of_nazareth_belfast/ m4_d94_transcript_red_opt.pdf, p. 23 Retrieved 10 June 2016

29. www.iicsa.org.uk/news/independent-inquiry-into-child-sexu-al-abuse-announces-first-investigations Retrieved 1 September 2016

30. www.theguardian.com/uk-news/2016/may/19/child-sex-abuse-po-lice-expect-30000-goddard-inquiry-cases Retrieved 10 June 2016

31. www.thetimes.co.uk/article/child-abuse-inquiry-out-of-control-warns-judge-8x3j9gcfc Retrieved 7 September 2016

32. www.bbc.co.uk/news/uk-scotland-36706790 Retrieved 4 July 2016

33. Proctor, Cohen, and Galloway, 2016

34. Diocese of Rochester, 2016

Chapter 23: A Future for Children's Homes?

1. Berridge and Brodie, Children's Homes Revisted, 1998

2. Department of Health, 1991

3. Narey, 2016, p. 6

4. Department for Education, 2014, p. 4

5. Ofsted, 2015, p. 39

6. Narey, 2016

7. *Ibid.*, pp. 6-7

8. Ofsted, 2015, p. 41

9. Narey, 2016, pp. 55-56

10. *Ibid.*, p. 21

11. *Ibid.*, p. 22

12. Department for Education, 2014, p. 47

13. Narey, 2016, pp. 12-13
14. http://ww.linkmaker.co.uk
15. Ofsted, 2015, pp. 16-17
16. Department for Education, 2014, p. 25
17. Narey, 2016, pp. 18-19
18. *Ibid*, p.27
19. *Ibid.*, p. 18
20. *Ibid.*, p. 45
21. *Ibid.*, p. 46
22. *Ibid*, pp. 62-63
23. *Ibid.*, p. 69

Acknowledgement

This work contains public sector information licensed under the Open Government Licence v3.0.

Bibliography

Advisory Council on Child Care. (1970). Care and Treatment in a Planned Environment. London: HMSO.

Anonymous [Rudolf, E. d.]. (1922). The First Forty Years: a Chronicle of the Church of England Waifs and Strays Society 1881–1920. London: Church of England Waifs and Strays Society / SPCK.

Anonymous. (1818). An Account of the School for the Indigent Blind in St. George's Fields. London.

Anonymous. (1960). Prisons and Borstals. London: HMSO.

Anonymous. (n.d.). Early History of Shaftesbury Homes & Arethusa. Retrieved 10 June 10, 2016, from TS Arethusa Old Boys' Association: http://www.ts_arethusa.talktalk.net/index_files/Page829.htm

Ashby, R. (2013). The History of TACT. The Actors' Children's Trust. Retrieved 21 November 2013, from http://www.tactactors.org/pdf/History%20 of%20TACT.pdf

Ayers, G. M. (1971). England's First State Hospitals 1867-1930. London: Wellcome Institute of the History of Medicine.

Bailey, M. (1996). The Chance of a Lifetime: The Shaftesbury Homes and Arethusa – 150 Years. Cirencester: Dianthus Publishing.

Barnardo, S. and Merchant, J. (1907). Memoirs of the Late Dr Barnardo. London: Hodder and Stoughton.

Barnett, M. G. (1913). Young Delinquents. A study of reformatory and industrial schools. London: Methuen.

Barritt, G. E. (1972). The Edgworth Story. London: National Children's Home.

Bartley, P. (2000). Prostitution: Prevention and Reform in England, 1860–1914. London: Routledge.

Berridge, D. (1985). Children's Homes. Oxford: Basil Blackwell.

Berridge, D. and Brodie, I. (1998). Children's Homes Revisited. London: Jessica Kingsley.

Birmingham City Council Children's Department. (1953). The First Four Years. Birmingham: Birmingham City Council.

Birt, L. M. (1913). The Children's Home-Finder: the story of Annie Macpherson and Louisa Birt. London: J. Nisbet.

Boyd, D. (1986). The Gordon Heritage (1885–1985). London: Robert Hale.

Bradfield, W. (1913). The Life of the Reverend Thomas Bowman Stephenson. London: Charles H. Kelly.

Care of Children Committee. (1946). Report of the Care of Children Committee. London: HMSO.

Carradice, P. (2009). Nautical Training Ships. Stroud: Amberley Publishing.

Chaplin, C. (1979). My Early Years. London: Bodley Head.

Charity Organisation Society. (1890). The Charities Register and Digest. London: Longmans, Green & Co.

Charity Organisation Society. (1893). The Epileptic and Crippled Child and Adult. London: Swan Sonnenschein & Co.

Charity Organisation Society. (1939). Annual Register of Charities and Public Institutions. London: Longmans & Co.

City of Manchester Children's Committee. (1956). Annual Report 1955-56. Manchester: City of Manchester.

Cliffe, D. and Berridge, D. (1991). Closing Children's Homes. London: National Children's Bureau.

Crompton, F. (1997). Workhouse Children: Infant and Child Paupers under the Worcestershire Poor Law, 1780-1871. Stroud: Sutton.

Cummings, L. (2008). Forgotten. London: Pan Books.

Curnock, N. (1901). The Story of the Children's Home. London: C. H. Kelly.

Cuthbert, V. (1937). Where Dreams Come True: A Record of 95 Years. London: Shaftesbury Homes.

Danczuk, S. (2014). Smile for the Camera: The Double Life of Cyril Smith. London: Biteback Publishing.

Department for Education. (2014). Children's Homes Data Pack. London: HMG.

Department of Health. (1991). Children Act Guidance and Regulations Volume 4: Residential Care. London: 1991 The Stationery Office.

Dickens, C. (1851). 'Lambs to be Fed'. Household Words, August 30, pp. 544-549.

Diocese of Rochester. (July 13 2016). Kendall House Review Press Conference Statements. Retrieved 14 July 2016, from Diocese of Rochester: http://www.rochester.anglican.org/content/pages/documents/1468411255.pdf

Duckworth, J. S. (1995). The Hardwicke Reformatory School, Gloucestershire. Transactions of the Bristol and Gloucestershire Archaeological Society, 113, 151-165.

Finnigan, R. (2013). 150th Anniversary History 1863-2013 Catholic Care, Diocese of Leeds. Leeds: Catholic Care.

Fletcher, W. (2005). Keeping the Vision Alive: the story of Barnardo's 1905-2005. Barkingside, Essex: Barnardo's.

Fox, L. W. (1952). The English Prison and Borstal Systems. London: Routledge & Kegan Paul.

Fullerton, W. Y. (1930). J.W.C. Fegan: A Tribute. London: Marshall, Morgan & Scott.

Furnival, J. (2005). Children of the Second Spring: Father James Nugent and the Work of Childcare in Liverpool. Leominster: Gracewing.

Gilbert, W. (1872). The Idiot Colony at Caterham. Good Words, 271-277.

Gillard, D. (2011). Education in England: a brief history. Retrieved 10 June 2016, from http://www.educationengland.org.uk/history/chapter02. html

Glen, W. C. (1879). The Poor Law Orders. London: Shaw and Sons.

Gray-Wilson, S. (2000). It Isn't Always Raining. Dalbeattie.

Guthrie, T. (1849). 'A Second Plea for Ragged Schools; or, Prevention Better than Cure'. The North British Review, p. 76.

Hamblin, A. (2010). If Only These Walls Could Speak. Codicote, Hertfordshire: Blenheim Press.

Havers, M. (2006). The Reformatory at Mount St Bernard Abbey 1856-1881. Coalville: Mount St Bernard Abbey.

Heath-Stubbs, M. (1935). Friendship's Highway: Being the History of the Girls' Friendly Society 1875–1935. London: Girls' Friendly Society.

Hicks, J. D. (1996). The Yorkshire Catholic Reformatory, Market Weighton. Beverley: East Yorkshire Local History Society.

Higginbotham, P. (2008). The Workhouse Cookbook. Stroud: The History Press.

Higginbotham, P. (2010). The Prison Cookbook. Stroud: The History Press.

Higginbotham, P. (2012). The Workhouse Encyclopedia. Stroud: The History Press.

Hitchman, J. (1966). They Carried the Sword. London: Gollancz.

Home Office. (1951). Sixth Report on the Work of the Children's Department. London: HMSO.

Hughson, D. (1807). London; being an accurate history and description of the British metropolis and its neighbourhood (Vol. 4). London: J. Stratford.

Hyland, J. (1993). Yesterday's Answers: Development and Decline of Schools for Young Offenders. London: Whiting & Birch.

Hyland, J. (2009). Changing Times Changing Needs: A History of the Catholic Children's Society (Westminster). London: Catholic Children's Society (Westminster).

Jacka, A. (1969). The Story of the Children's Home 1869–1969. Harpenden: National Children's Home.

Jeffs, E. (1930). Motherless: the story of Robert Thomson Smith and the first homes for motherless children. London: Marshall, Morgan and Scott.

Jillings, J. (1996). Child Abuse: An independent investigation commissioned by Clwyd County Council 1974–1995.

Jones, K. (1972). A History of the Mental Health Services. London: Routledge & Kegan Paul.

Jones, M. G. (1938). The Charity School Movement: A Study in Eighteenth Century Puritanism in Action. Cambridge: CUP.

Kirkwood, A. (1992). The Leicestershire Inquiry.

Kohli, M. (2003). The Golden Bridge: Young Immigrants to Canada 1833–1939. Toronto: Natural Heritage Books.

Kohli, M. (2016). William John Pady. The British Home Child, 6(2).

Lacey, P., Ashdown, R., Jones, P., Lawson, H. and Pipe, M. (Eds.). (2015). The Routledge Companion to Severe, Profound and Multiple Learning Difficulties. London: Routledge.

Lawson, J. and Silver, H. (1973). A Social History of Education in England. London: Methuen.

Leonard, E. M. (1900). The Early History of English Poor Relief. Cambridge: Cambridge University Press.

Levy, A. and Kahan, B. (1990). The Pindown Experience and the Protection of Children. Staffordshire County Council.

Lynch, D. (1982). Chariots of the Gospel. The Centenary History of the Church Army. Worthing: H. E. Walter.

Maddison, A. J. (1898). Hints on Rescue Work. London: Reformatory and Refuge Union.

Magnusson, A. (2006). The Quarrier's Story: A History of Quarriers. Edinburgh: Dundurn / Birlinn.

Mahood, L. (1990). The Magdalenes. London: Routledge.

Manzione, C. K. (1995). Christ's Hospital of London, 1552-1598: A Passing Deed of Pity. Susquehanna University Press.

Martin, N. (1983). A Man with a Vision: the Story of John Groom. Exeter: Religious and Moral Education Press.

McConville, S. (1981). A History of English Prison Administration. London: Routledge & Kegan Paul.

McDougall, A. and Plant, W. A. (1913). Schools for Epileptics, and the Education of Epileptic Children in England. Epilepsia, 358-361.

Morris, L. (2011). The Violets Are Mine: Tales of an Unwanted Orphan. Xlibris Corporation.

Narey, S. M. (2016). Residential Care in England. London.

Nichols, R. H. and Wray, F. A. (1935). The History of the Foundling Hospital. Oxford: Oxford University Press.

Nokes, H. (1886). Twenty-Three Years in a House of Mercy. London: Rivingtons.

O'Hara, M. (3 June 2015). Children's Care Homes supplement. The Guardian.

Ofsted. (2015). Children looked after placement data. London: HMG.

Oldfield, S. (2008). Jeanie, an 'Army of One': Mrs Nassau Senior 1828–1877 The First Woman in Whitehall. Brighton: Sussex Academic Press.

Oswin, M. (1975). Handicapped children and the 'hospital scandal reports'. Child: Care, Health and Development, 1, 71-77.

Parker, R. (1990). Away from Home: a history of child care. Barkingside, Essex: Barnardo's.

Parker, R. (2010). Uprooted: The Shipment of Poor Children to Canada, 1867–1917. Bristol: Policy Press.

Parker, R. (2015). Change and Continuity in Children's Services. Bristol: Policy Press.

Partington, C. F. (1834). National History and Views of London and Its Environs: Vol. II. London: Simpkin & Marshall.

Pearce, S. B. (1958). An Ideal in the Working. London: The Magdalen Hospital.

Pearl, V. (1978). Puritans and Poor Relief: The London Workhouse, 1649–1660. In K. Thomas and D. Pennington, Puritans and Revolutionaries (pp. 206-232). London: Clarendon Press.

Philpot, T. (1994). Action for Children. Oxford: Lion.

Philpott, H. B. (1904). London at School: the Story of the School Board. London: Fisher Unwin.

Pinchbeck, I. and Hewitt, M. (1973). Children in English Society Volume. II: From the Eighteenth Century to the Children Act 1948. London: Routledge and Kegan Paul.

Pinches, S. M. (1998). Father Hudson and His Society: A History 1898–1998. Birmingham: Archdiocese of Birmingham Historical Commission.

Prahms, W. (2006). Newcastle Ragged and Industrial School. Stroud: The History Press.

Proctor, S., Cohen, S. and Galloway, R. (2016, June). Report of a Review of Kendall House, Gravesend 1967–1986. Retrieved 14 July 2016, from Diocese of Rochester: http://www.rochester.anglican.org/content/pages/documents/1468406891.pdf

Pugh, G. (2011). London's Forgotten Children: Thomas Coram and the Foundling Hospital. Stroud: The History Press.

Ray, C. (1903). The Life of Charles Haddon Spurgeon. London: Isbister.

Reformatory and Refuge Union. (1912). Classified List of Child-Saving Institutions. London: Reformatory and Refuge Union.

Richardson, H. (1998). English Hospitals 1660–1948. Swindon: RCHME.

Rimmer, J. (1986). Yesterday's Naughty Children. Manchester: Neil Richardson.

Rose, J. (1987). For the Sake of the Children. London: Hodder & Stoughton.

Russell, C. E. (1906). The Making of the Criminal. London: Macmillan.

Ryan, S. (2009). Executive Summary. Retrieved 10 June 2016, from The Commission to Inquire into Child Abuse: http://www.childabusecommission.ie/rpt/pdfs/CICA-Executive%20Summary.pdf

Rye, M. (1870). First Report of the Placing Out of Pauper and Other Orphans in Canada and the United States of America. London.

Sandall, R., Wiggins, A. R. and Coutts, F. L. (1955). The History of the Salvation Army: 1883–1953 Social Reform and Welfare Work. Edinburgh: T. Nelson.

Scottish Home Department. (1946). Report of the Committee on Homeless Children. Edinburgh: HMSO.

Sisters of Nazareth. (2016). Brief History of the Sisters of Nazareth. Retrieved 26 May 2016, from www.sistersofnazareth.com/brief-history-of-the-sisters-of-nazareth

Slocombe, I. (2005). Wiltshire Reformatory for Boys, Warminster, 1856-1924. East Knoyle: Hobnob Press.

Smart, C. (2000). Reconsidering the Recent History of Child Sexual Abuse, 1910–1960. Journal of Social Policy, 29, 55-71.

Smithers, H. (1825). Liverpool, its commerce, statistics and institutions: with a history of the cotton trade. Liverpool: T. Kaye.

Stoke Park Hospital – the Latter Years (n.d.). [Motion Picture]. Retrieved 10 June 2016, from Bristol Stories: http://www.bristolstories.org/story/195

Stroud, J. (1971). Thirteen Penny Stamps: The Story of the Church of England Children's Society from its Beginnings as 'Waifs and Strays'. London: Hodder & Stoughton.

Strype, J. (1720). A Survey of the Cities of London and Westminster, Vol. 1.

Tayler, W. E. (1871). The Bristol Orphan Houses. London: Morgan and Scott.

Taylor, W. J. (1907). The Story of the Homes. Being a record of their origin, development and work for fifty years. London: London Female Preventive and Reformatory Institution.

Trimmer, S. (1792). Reflections upon the Education of Children in Charity Schools. London: Longman.

Urey, G. (1985). The Newton Hall Story: 80 Years of Caring. Frodsham: National Children's Home.

Utting, W. B. (1991). Children in Public Care: a review of residential child care. London: HMSO.

Wagner, G. (1979). Barnardo. London: Weidenfeld & Nicholson.

Wagner, G. (1982). Children of the Empire. London: Weidenfeld & Nicolson.

Walpole, C. F. (1941). Golden Links. London: Epworth Press.

Warner, N. (1992). Choosing with Care: the Report of the Committee of Inquiry into the Selection, Development and Management of Staff in Children's Homes. London: HMSO.

Warren, M. (2013). James Dixon's Children: The Story of Blackburn Orphanage. Lancaster: Fleetfoot Books.

Waterhouse, R. (1999). Lost in Care: Report of the Tribunal of Inquiry into the Abuse of Children in Care in the Former County Council Areas of Gwynedd and Clwyd since 1974. The Stationery Office.

Waugh, N. (1911). These, My Little Ones. London: Sands & Co.

Williams, A. E. (1943). Barnardo of Stepney, the Father of Nobody's Children. London: George Allen & Unwin.

Wolff, M. (1967). Prison. London: Eyre & Spottiswoode.

Women's Group on Public Welfare. (1943). Our Towns: A Close-Up. London: Oxford University Press.

Wythen Baxter, G. R. (1841). The Book of the Bastiles. London: John Stephens.

Index